A Simple and Practical Handbook Of Achieving Optimal Health Through Good Digestion.

UNLIMITED HEALTH

by

Dr. Douglas Lobay, N.D.

A Modern and Scientific Guide to the Use of Food, Nutrition and Diet Therapy.

Published by
Apple Communications
Kelowna, B.C.

Disclaimer: The information presented here in this book is for educational purposes only and is not intended as a substitute for proper medical care. Individuals should seek out proper medical care from licensed health care practitioners for appropriate diagnosis and treatment.

Canadian Cataloguing in Publication Data
Lobay, Doug, 1965 -
Unlimited Health

Includes Index
ISBN: 0-9695681-1-8
1. Naturopathy - Handbooks, manuals, etc. 2. Diet - Natural
3. Digestion and Disease
I. Title RZ 430.173 1994
615.5'35" 94-10653

Printed in the United States of America

Acknowledgements

I would like to thank:

Mom and Dad
Arlene and Jim
Mike and Annette
Mike and Nellie
Dr. Jonn Matsen
Dr. Gaetano Morello
Dr. Garrett Swetlikoff
Dr. Kim Vanderlinden
and of course, Natalie

Dedication

To Natalie for all her love and support.

A Different Drummer

"Why should we be in such desperate haste to succeed and in such desperate enterprises? If a man does not keep pace with his companions, perhaps it is because he hears a different drummer. Let him step to the music he hears, however measured or far away. It is not important that he should mature as soon as an apple tree or oak. However mean your life is, meet it and live it; do not shun it and call it hard names. It is not so bad as you are. It looks poorest when you are richest. The fault-finder will find faults even in paradise. Love your life, poor as it is. You may perhaps have some pleasant, thrilling, glorious hours, even in a poorhouse. The setting sun is reflected from the windows of the almshouse as brightly as from the rich man's abode. Cultivate poverty like a garden herb like sage. Do not trouble yourself much to get new things, whether clothes or friends. Turn the old; return to them. Things do not change; we change. Sell your clothes and keep your thoughts. God will see that you do not want society. It is life near the bone where it is sweetest. Superfluous wealth can buy superfluities only. Money is not required to buy one necessary of the soul."

Henry David Thoreau

Table of Contents

Preface

The purpose of "Unlimited Health" is to provide a modern and scientific guide to the use of diet and digestion in achieving optimal health. I wanted to present a simple and practical handbook designed to educate others on the virtues of good digestion and a healthy diet. The trouble with so many of the diet books in circulation today is that they are confusing, contradictory and impractical. Diet should be simple and easy to follow. It should be straight forward and practical. Good digestion, natural foods and the practical principles of food combining are necessary for achieving optimal health.

After graduating from naturopathic medical college in Seattle, Washington in 1991 my mind was inundated with medical facts and figures. In school I thought I had learned all the medical information necessary to cure most disease. I had studied the Merck Manual and other medical textbooks from cover to cover. However, I soon realized I was short on practical experience. Rather than start my own medical practice I was asked to join a busy naturopathic office in North Vancouver. I was fortunate to have the opportunity to work at an established naturopathic clinic with some eminent naturopathic physicians. The focus of the clinic was the use diet and digestion to treat disease. However, at this point I was interested in high tech naturopathic medicine, not diet and digestion. I had some difficulty in adjusting the focus of treatment from high tech pursuits to simple aspects of diet and nutrition. But I finally got the message and came to the realization that simple dietary and lifestyle changes can make significant improvement in a person's state of health.

When I first started writing about natural medicine my work was complex, scientific and confusing. I had to prove to myself that there was a scientific explanation to the therapies and treatments that naturopathic physicians employ. The first book I wrote was a culmination of this scientific research and a desire to communicate to the lay person. The book was virtual cookbook of using different vitamins, minerals, food supplements and herbal medicines to treat disease. After gaining several years of practical experience my approach to writing has softened. I wanted to write material that was simple, practical and easily digestible. I decided that the focus of my next book would be about foods, nutrition and digestion. I didn't want to even mention vitamins and minerals. I wanted to write a simple and practical guide that would be easy to read and just as easy to follow. The results of my labour is "Unlimited Health."

"Unlimited Health" is designed to be a simple and practical handbook of using food, nutrition and diet therapy. I first explain the process of digestion, maldigestion and modern disease. Good health begins with good digestion. Knowing the principles of good digestion are imperative for unlimited health. I further explain the connection between health and the immune system and the glandular system. In the next part of the book I discuss the connection between specific modern foods and disease. I further discuss the health benefits of natural foods. The third part of this book focuses on a dietary program designed to achieve optimal health. I briefly discuss the connection between the state of your blood and your health. I further explain the principles of a healthy diet and food combining. The last part of the book outlines menu suggestions and lists over one hundred of my favorite recipes.

I challenge you make a change in your life that can impact your health. Make a simple change, whether it is cutting out your coffee, decreasing your sugar consumption, avoiding excess fats, following the principles of food combining or changing the way you eat. You can make these changes and you can change your health and the way you feel. You can achieve unlimited health.

Doug Lobay,

Kelowna, B.C.

Introduction

I am often reminded of the quotation by the American inventor Thomas A. Edison. He said and I quote "The doctor of the future will give no medicine, but will interest their patients in the care of the human frame, in proper diet and in cause and prevention of disease." The ancient scientist and philosopher Hippocrates always said, "Let your food be your medicine and your medicine be your food." The connection between food, diet and disease has been recognized for thousands of years. We are now rediscovering this important connection and its impact on your health. What you eat and how you eat it can influence the way you feel and live.

All chronic disease begins with poor digestion. There is a strong connection between disease and diet. Scientific research is now beginning to catch up and validate this important relationship. Naturopathic physicians have long preached the virtues of a natural diet, good nutrition and optimal health. A poor diet results in poor digestion and ill health. The modern fast food diet rich in caffeine, fats, salt, sugar, additives and preservatives results in ill health. A natural diet rich in whole grains and cereals, fresh fruits and vegetables contributes to good digestion and optimal health. This book serves as a guide to using food, diet and nutrition in achieving better health. We all can make changes in some aspect of our diet including the foods we eat and how we eat them.

What is health? What is good health? What is optimal health? Health is defined in Webster's dictionary as a state of physical, mental and social well being. Health is not merely a condition of being disease free. Health is a condition of physical, mental, social and spiritual well being. Good health is a condition of good physical, mental, social and spiritual well being. Optimal health is a condition of optimal physical, mental, social and spiritual well being. Unlimited health is achieved by removing the limiting factors that prevents a person from achieving optimal health. Food, diet and nutrition are limiting factors in achieving optimal health.

Modern medicine focuses on a disease oriented model of health. The modern medical establishment contends that health is a result of being disease free. Ill-health results when an organism is traumatized by disease. Their primary focus is on physical disease and to a lesser extent on mental disease. Modern medicine works very well in treating acute disease and trauma, but falls short in treating chronic disease and getting people healthy. If you break a bone modern medicine works very well in resetting the bone and helping to prevent infection. However, it does very little in optimizing the healing process and helping the patient reach optimal health. A person who has a recurrent sore throat is often prescribed antibiotics or analgesics to help prevent the associated pain or discomfort. There is often little discussion in terms of prevention. There is no discussion about the immune system and factors that can impair or stimulate immune function. The doctor seldom discusses diet, nutrition, personal hygiene and nutrients that can help improve the state of health of the individual. If you want cure acute disease go to a medical doctor. If you want to heal yourself and get healthy go to a naturopathic physician. There must be a shift from the disease oriented model of health to a holistic model of health that incorporates the physical, mental, social and spiritual aspects of health.

Holistic health is a system of preventive medicine that takes into account the whole individual, their own responsibility for their well-being and the total influences including social, psychological and environmental factors. Holistic health addresses aspects of lifestyle, diet, nutrition and their impact on overall well being. Food, nutrition and diet play an important role in holistic health. What we eat, how and when we eat it can influence our overall well being.

The human body is incredibly complex and interrelated. One area or organ in the body can have a strong influence on another area or organ. Mental, emotional and spiritual state can influence the physical state. When a person is happy their entire being radiates happiness. Not only their emotional state is happy but also their physical, mental and spiritual state. Their heart is happy, their brain and nervous system is happy and their digestive system is happy. Happy hormones are produced in the brain, nervous system and various glands throughout the body. Conversely, when a person is sick their whole being radiates sickness. The human body has an inherent healing process that maintains and restores health. Naturopathic physicians work to restore and support these inherent healing systems when they have broken down, by using methods, medicines and techniques that are in harmony with natural processes. Natural foods and good nutrition can stimulate the inherent healing process within the human body. Natural foods can truly be a healing medicine.

Digestion plays an important role in overall health. Good digestion, in addition to good food and good nutrition, is required for achieving optimal health. In our fast paced, secular lifestyle we tend to eat too fast, eat under stress and eat too many poorly combined foods. This places extreme demands on our digestive system. Modern diseases that affect the digestive system include heartburn, hiatus hernia, peptic ulcers, gallstones, colitis, irritable bowel syndrome, constipation and diverticulosis. Other diseases such as diabetes, gout, eczema and even cancer result from poor digestion. We can improve our digestion by eating good, wholesome natural foods and adhering to the principles of proper food combining.

Food, nutrition and diet therapy are an important cornerstone of modern naturopathic medicine. Chronic, degenerative disease is caused by modern, refined and processed foods, bad nutrition and poor diet. This book serves as a simple and practical guide of achieving optimal health through natural foods, good nutrition and good digestion. You can be healthier by eating better. If you are sick or have disease you can help stimulate your inherent healing processes by eating better. Remember the old adage, "An apple a day keeps the doctor away." Follow the principles outlined in this book and you can achieve unlimited health.

PART I

Digestion, Disease and Health

1

The Mouth and Esophagus

The mouth is the opening that forms the beginning of the digestive system. Teeth in the mouth help to break large food particles into smaller particles. The mouth is a major organ of speech and emotional expression. The mouth is also the site of the organs of taste. The esophagus is a hollow tube that connects the mouth to the stomach.

Tongue

The tongue is a muscular organ on the floor of the mouth that aids in chewing, swallowing and speech. The tongue is also the organ of taste for the human body. In oriental medicine tongue analysis is commonly used to help diagnose disease. A normal tongue is a full, slightly damp, red organ with a slight white coating. However, most people in western countries have a tongue with a thick, damp white coating. A tongue with a thick, damp, white coating represents too much dampness in the interior of the body. The most common cause of this condition is a diet rich in sugar, refined carbohydrates and processed foods. In oriental medicine the tongue represents a window to the heart. A pale, dull tongue represents a lack of energy in the heart. A thick, red, flabby tongue represents too much energy in the heart. A dry, cracked tongue represents diminished energy in the heart.

Taste

Taste is the peculiar sensation perceived from the contact of food and fluid with the tongue. Taste represents a complex interplay between foods and fluids with taste buds and the nerves they are connected to. Taste buds are bundles of slender cells with hair-like branches that are packed together to form papillae on the upper surface of the tongue.

When substance enters the mouth molecules enter the pores in the papillae and stimulate the sensation of taste. In order for a substance to does this it must be dissolved in liquid. If it is not dissolved in liquid then it must be broken down, melted, chewed and mixed with saliva.

There are four basic tastes: sweet, sour, salty and bitter. All other tastes are combinations of these basic tastes. Sometimes alkaline and metallic are included as distinct taste. The taste buds are specialized and respond to one distinct taste. The sweet and salty taste buds are located in the tip and front part of the tongue. Sour taste buds are located mainly along the sides of the tongue. Bitter taste buds are mainly located at the back of the tongue. The solid center of the tongue has very few taste buds.

The trouble with taste buds is that they can alter our mood and behavior. Taste buds have a direct connection to a part of the brain called the limbic system. The limbic system is the part of the brain that controls certain aspects of mood and behavior. The limbic system produces chemicals that can cause feelings of pleasure and euphoria. Highly addictive chemicals such as endorphins and enkephalins can produce these feelings. Certain foods can stimulate nerves in the taste buds that consequently stimulate nerves in the limbic system to produce these highly addictive chemicals. Sugar is a prime example of a food that is highly addictive. Sugar tastes good and it makes us feel good when we're eating it. A high consumption of sugar sensitizes our taste buds. This partially explains why we consume so much sugar.

Salivary Glands

Salivary glands refer to any glands in the mouth that contribute to the production of saliva. There are three major pairs of salivary glands including the parotid, submaxillary and sublingual glands. There are thousands of other small salivary glands within the cheeks and and on the tongue.

The parotid glands are the largest salivary glands and are located directly in front of and below the ears at the angle of the jaw. Saliva produced in the parotid glands travels across the cheeks in a hollow tube called Stenson's duct. The submaxillary glands are located underneath and inside the jaw and discharge saliva upwards through a small duct that enters at the floor of the mouth. The sublingual glands are located below and underneath the tongue and discharge saliva upwards into the floor of the mouth.

Saliva is needed to moisten the mouth, lubricate food and make swallowing easier. Saliva also contains the enzyme ptyalin. Ptyalin breaks down large starch molecules into smaller chunks. Salivary glands produce an enormous amount of fluid on a daily basis. The daily production of saliva ranges between 0.8 and 1.5 liters of fluid per day. Saliva is slightly acidic and has a pH between 6.0 and 7.4.

Saliva is composed of water, minerals, proteins and enzymes. Saliva contains up to 97% water by weight. Saliva contains many minerals especially large quantities of potassium and bicarbonate ions. Saliva contains mucous, a mixture of different proteins including mucin, that helps to lubricate foods and make swallowing easier. Saliva also contains several enzymes including ptyalin that begins to digest starches.

Saliva plays a very important role in maintaining good oral hygiene. The mouth is load with bacteria that can cause inflammation and cavities. The flow of saliva helps to wash away bacteria. Saliva also contains natural antibiotics that actually destroy bacteria. In the absence of salivation the mouth becomes ulcerated and otherwise infected and tooth decay becomes rampant˙

The salivary glands are controlled by the nervous system. The production of saliva can he stimulated by the site, taste or smell of food. It only takes two to three seconds from appearance of food to stimulate the release of saliva. This quick response is an automatic reflex.

Excess Saliva

Occasionally, the salivary glands produce too much saliva. Excess saliva may be caused by many conditions including local irritation in the mouth, poor fitting dental appliances, disturbances of digestion including acid reflux from the stomach, abnormalities of the nervous system and increased consumption of starches and simple sugars. A diet rich in sugar and refined carbohydrates stimulates the salivary glands to produce too much saliva.

Decreased Saliva

Decreased production of saliva is otherwise known as a dry mouth and is much more common than excess saliva. Decreased production of saliva is a normal process of aging. Production of salivary fluid can decrease 40 to 60% of normal volume with advanced age. Dehydration frequently decreases the production of saliva in an effort to conserve water and minerals. Certain illnesses including mumps; an infection of the parotid glands, sarcoidosis and Sjogren's disease can produce a dry mouth. Trauma or infection to the nervous system can decrease saliva production. Morphine, atropine and other similar drugs can produce a marked decrease in the amount of saliva. Nutritional deficiencies of potassium and the vitamin B-complex family including vitamin B1, B2 and B12 can decrease the production of saliva and result in a dry mouth. All sweet and bitter foods stimulate the salivary glands to produce saliva.

Salivary Gland Obstruction

An obstruction of the duct leading from the salivary gland to the mouth can occur. Salivary fluid backs up and leads to an abnormal enlargement of the gland. The parotid and the submaxillary glands are usually affected while the sublingual glands are almost never affected. The most common cause of salivary gland obstruction is by a calcium stone that rarely exceeds the size of a kernel of rice. The calcium stone may become lodged in the salivary duct. The resulting obstruction to the gland may or may not be painful and may become unsightly if is allowed to be untreated. Many simple stones can be manually expressed by repeatedly pressing your fingers of the duct or by applying a hot compress to the gland to help dilate the duct. Another method is to acidify the mouth and glands in an effort to dissolve the alkaline calcium stone.

Canker Sores

Canker sores are acute, painful ulcerations, less that one centimeter in diameter that occur on the lips, gums and mouth of an affected individual. Canker sores have white centers and are surrounded by red, inflammed borders. These ulcerations may be painful. They tend to localize on the inner and outer lips, the outer gums and the inside of the mouth.

Canker sores are estimated to affect 20% of the North American population. They occur more commonly in females than in males. Canker sores usually occur as multiple, small little ulcerations that are painful. These sores usually heal spontaneously within 10 to 14 days, but they have a high tendency to recur. Exacerbations and remissions throughout life are common. Stress and food allergies are the two most common causes of canker sores. Stressful conditions can frequently precipitate canker sores. Common foods that trigger canker sores include citrus fruits, milk, sugar, chocolate, peanuts and wheat. Canker sores heal spontaneously after the stressful condition or offending food is removed from the diet.

Tonsils

Tonsils are small, rounded masses of lymph tissue that help to filter out bacteria and other foreign material that may enter the body, especially through the mouth and nose. There are three different types of tonsils. The structures usually referred to as tonsils are the palatine tonsils. The palatine tonsils are a pair of lymph glands about the size of almonds located on either side at the back of the throat. Below them at the base of the tongue are the lingual tonsils. On the upper rear wall of the throat are the pharyngeal or adenoid tonsils. Tonsils are the first line of defence by the immune system of bacteria and foreign material that enters the body through the mouth and nose. Tonsils can get clogged up from poor diet, poor lymphatic drainage and poor immune system function.

Tonsillitis

Tonsillitis is an inflammation and enlargement of a tonsil, especially the palatine tonsils located at the back of the throat. Enlarged tonsils need not be a concern unless they become chronically infected and interfere with swallowing and breathing. They may become enlarged in the process of filtering frequent, minor infections. The adenoids usually grow larger in children until the age of five years and then they may cease to become troublesome. One more serious form of tonsillitis is caused by streptococcal bacteria infection of the throat. A excess consumption of mucous forming foods can clog up the tonsils and impair their ability to filter toxins.

Esophagus

The esophagus is a narrow, muscular tube that connects the mouth to the stomach. The function of the esophagus is to conduct food and fluids from the mouth to the stomach and prevent reflux of stomach contents into the esophagus. The esophagus is approximately 30 centimeters or 12 inches long and passes through the chest through the diaphragm into the stomach. The junction between the stomach and esophagus is closed by a muscular valve known as the cardiac valve. This cardiac valve opens to allow the passage of food into the stomach and prevents reflux of food from the stomach back into the esophagus. Disorders of the esophagus often involve either an obstruction or a reflux of food or stomach juice. The inner lining of the esophagus produces large amounts of mucous that helps to prevent any irritation from swallowed food or any reflux of stomach contents. Inflammation of the esophagus usually occurs when the highly acid stomach contents reflux up into the esophagus.

Peristalsis

When food is swallowed it passes into the esophagus. Strong, muscular contractions in the walls of esophagus occur to help propel food down to the stomach. The rhythmical, wave-like contractions of these muscles is called peristalsis. The peristaltic contractions also help to propel food forward in the stomach and intestines. Peristalsis also helps to mix food and aids in its break down and digestion. Stress can impair these muscle and prevent normal muscular contractions.

Globus Hystericus

Globus hystericus is the term used to describe the abnormal sensation of a mass or lump in the back of the throat. However, no real mass or lump is present. Globus hystericus is frequently caused by emotional stress and tension. Unlike other physical blockages in the upper esophagus this globus sensation is not affected by swallowing and is not relieved with drinking fluids. This sensation often disappears with time after the emotional stressors have been relieved.

Esophageal Obstruction

A failure of the cardiac sphincter to open when swallowing food results in esophageal obstruction. The cause of esophageal obstruction is unkown but anxiety and emotional tension seem to aggravate this condition and precipitate attacks. As this condition progresses there may an abnormal dilation of the esophagus and a loss of normal peristaltic contractions. An individual with esophageal obstruction complains of difficulty swallowing, feeling of fulness in the chest and vomiting frequently occurs. Large meals should be avoided and all meals should be eaten slowly with frequent drinking of fluids. Aromatic oils from chamomile, ginger, lemon balm and peppermint help to relax the cardiac sphincter.

Heartburn

Heartburn really has nothing to do with the heart but rather due to inflammation of the esophagus. Heartburn is the term used to describe the burning sensation that can occur as a result of reflux of stomach contents into the esophagus. The normally thin, protective lining of the esophagus becomes severely irritated from reflux of the highly acidic stomach contents. Intense pain and burning often is experienced. Abnormal relaxation of the cardiac sphincter separating the esophagus and stomach can occur. Factors known to contribute abnormal relaxation of the cardiac sphincter include overindulgence in coffee, tea, sugar, chocolate, fried foods, alcohol and spicy foods.

Patient Files

Patricia M. was a 72 year old widow who came into our office complaining of a dry mouth, poor digestion and frequent heartburn. She had trouble swallowing food and complained of a constant lump in the back of the throat. She also complained of fatigue and lack of energy. A routine blood test revealed she was low in iron. A dietary review revealed poor eating habits. She lived alone and frequently consumed canned and processed foods. She seldom ate fresh fruits and vegetables. We made some simple dietary changes and suggested she consume of wider variety of foods including fresh fruits and vegetables. We prescribed digestive enzymes and bitters to help increase salivation and improve digestion. We also recommended iron, zinc and vitamin B-12 supplementation. After three weeks of following our instructions she indicated that she felt much better, she had more energy and her digestion was much improved.

Walter F. was a 42 year old teacher who came into our office complaining of recurrent painful, ulcerations on the inside of his lips, gums and inner mouth. Physical examination revealed small little ulcerations that resembled grains of salt surrounded by a red, raised border. We confirmed our suspicion that he had canker sores. We questioned him about his lifestyle and dietary habits. He indicated that he was under quite a bit of stress with work and family commitments. We told him that canker sores were frequently precipitated by stress. A dietary review revealed that he consumed large amounts of peanuts and citrus fruits. A food sensitivity test helped to identify allergic foods. He was told to avoid offending foods and make some simple dietary changes. After 3 months he had no outbreaks of canker sores and he also remarked he felt much better.

2

The Stomach

The stomach is a sensitive, little organ that plays a very important role in the digestive process. The stomach is also one of the most abused organs in the human body. Most people treat their stomach like a garbage disposal system. Food which resembles waste product is carelessly dumped into the stomach. Coffee, sugar, chocolate, white bread, donuts, french fries, alcohol and other refined and processed foods are dumped into the stomach. Most people consume a smorgasbord of foods at one meal. Large quantities of improperly combined foods are consumed and dumped in the stomach. The stomach literally goes into spasm. The beginning of poor digestion and ill health begins with poor stomach function.

The stomach is a curved, muscular sac-like structure that is between the esophagus and the small intestine. The stomach has four layers of muscle that account for the stomach's ability to expand when food enters it. When the stomach is empty it practically has no cavity at all and its walls are pressed tightly together. When full the average stomach holds about two liters of food and fluid.

Stomach Functions

The major functions of the stomach are to store, mix and digest food. The stomach stores food and only releases food when it can be accomodated in the lower portion of the digestive system. The stomach is responsible for mixing of food and fluid with stomach secretions until it forms a thick soup called chyme. The stomach also allows for the slow emptying of food into the small intestine at a rate suitable for proper digestion and absorption by the intestines. The stomach produces a large quantity of stomach secretions containing hydrochloric acid, enzymes and mucous. The stomach produces a daily volume of 1.5 liters of highly acidic fluid.

Hydrochloric Acid and Stomach Enzymes

Large quantities of hydrochloric acid are produced by stomach cells to digest protein in food. Hydrochloric acid breaks down large proteins into smaller chunks that are easily digested and absorbed in the small intestine. Stomach cells also produce a hormone called pepsin that further breaks down proteins. Small quantities of other enzymes are produced in the stomach including enzymes that breakdown starch and fats.

Intrinsic Factor

A substance called intrinsic factor, essential for absorption of vitamin B12 in the small intestine, is produced by the same cells that produce hydrochloric acid. Intrinsic factor is a small protein that binds to vitamin B12 and prevents its digestion in the stomach and enhances its absorption in the small intestine. Vitamin B12 is necessary for the development and maturation of red blood cells and the development of a healthy nervous system. Poor vitamin B12 absorption occurs in many individuals with poor stomach function.

Mucous

Mucous is a thick secretion composed mainly of water, minerals and several proteins containing large sugar molecules. Mucous is slightly different in different parts of the digestive system, but everywhere is has several important characteristics that make it both an excellent lubricant and a protectant for the wall of the gut. Mucous is produced in the stomach to help protect the lining of the stomach from the harmful effects of hydrochloric acid.

Peristalsis

When food enters the stomach the stomach muscle contract in rhythm. Their combined action sends a series of wave-like contractions from the upper end of the stomach to the lower end. These contractions known as peristalsis, mix the partially digested food and fluid with stomach secretions until it has the consistency of a thick soup. The muscle contractions then push the contents of the stomach into the beginning of the small intestine known as the duodenum.

Heartburn

Heartburn is the general term used to describe a burning sensation in the stomach. It has nothing to do with the heart at all except for the location of the discomfort. It is one of the most common signs of indigestion. Heartburn occurs when there is too much acid in the stomach or some of the acidic stomach contents travel up the esophagus. Poor dietary habits, improper food combining, excess consumption of spicy foods, refined and processed foods, sugar, chocolate, coffee, alcohol, excess consumption of hydrochloric acid and stress can cause heartburn.

The conventional treatment of heartburn is with antacids. Practically all of the over-the-counter antacids available contain at least one acid neutralizing substance. Common antacid ingredients include calcium carbonate, sodium bicarbonate, magnesium compounds and aluminum compounds. Calcium carbonate antacids including TUMS usually are effective for short term relief heartburn but can cause a rebound effect where stomach acid actually increases. Sodium bicarbonate can cause rebound gas and distention which may be equally uncomfortable. Large doses of sodium bicarbonate can upset the body's acid/base balance. Magnesium antacids including Milk of Magnesia can cause bloating and diarrhea in large doses. Aluminum compounds may cause constipation, especially in the elderly. With the recent connection of aluminum with Alzheimer's disease the consumption of aluminum based antacids is highly discouraged. Natural treatment of heartburn should be focused at identifing and eliminating prediposing factors and helping the stomach to relax and function better.

Decreased Stomach Acid

Hydrochloric production in the stomach decreases with age. It has been estimated that 50% of the people over the age of 60 years have low stomach acid levels. A lesser percentage of young adults also suffer from low stomach acid production. Symptoms of low stomach acid production include nausea, vomiting, bloating, beltching, indigestion, flatulence, burning in the stomach after meals, chronic yeast and other parasitic infections, undigested food particles in the stool, anal and rectal itching.

Diseases associated with low stomach acid production include alcoholism, asthma, eczema, psoriasis, acne, rosacea, chronic hives, vitiligo, chronic sinusitis, multiple food allergies, hypothyroidism, hyperthyroidism, hypoglycemia, diabetes, chronic auto-immune disorders, lupus, rheumatoid arthritis, sjogren's disease, liver disease, gall bladder disease, myasthenia gravis, osteoarthritis and osteoporosis. A type of anemia called pernicious anemia can develop. The same cells that produce hydrochloric acid also produce a small protein called intrinsic factor that helps to prevent the digestion of vitamin B12 in the stomach and enhance its absorption in the small intestine. When stomach acid production is low then intrinsic factor production is also low and anemia develops.

The best method for diagnosing low stomach is by the Heidelberg stomach analysis. A capsule containing a long string is swallowed shortly after eating. The capsule unravels as it travels from the mouth down the esophagus to the stomach. A small length of the string remains in the mouth so that the string may be retrieved after a period of time. The string in the capsule is pH sensitive and it turns different colours in the presence of different levels of acidity. After a period of time the string is retrieved by gently pulling the string from the mouth. The gelatin capsule is usually dissolved in the stomach and only the string remains. The colour of the portion of the string that was in the stomach is then compared to a standard chart of pH measurements.

Stomach Acidity Home Test

A simple home test for determining whether or not you have low stomach acid production can be performed with household vinegar, lemon juice or grapefruit juice. After you have eaten a meal, preferably high in protein, you can swallow two tablespoons of vinegar or other acid juice. If this makes your digestion better and your symptoms improve then you can be reasonably sure that you have low stomach acid production. However, if this makes your digestion worse and your symptoms get worse then you can be reasonably sure that your problem is too much stomach acid. If you observe no change in digestion and symptoms then you can repeat this experiment several times and increase the quantity of vinegar being consumed.

Stimulating Hydrochloric Acid Production

If you have been diagnosed with hypochlorhydria or low stomach acid production then you can help your stomach by naturally stimulating acid production. Bitters have been used medicinally for hundreds of years to help stimulate hydrochloric acid production. The consumption of a small amount of bitters before or with a meal will help to increase hydrochloric acid production and help digestion in the stomach.

Hydrochloric Acid Supplementation

If you have determined or have been diagnosed with low stomach acid production then you may need hydrochloric acid supplementation. Begin by taking one hydrochloric acid tablet or capsule containing 10 grains of hydrochloric acid at your next large meal, preferably a meal high in protein. Continue to increase the number of hydrochloric acid tablets or capsules by one at each meal until you feel a warmth or burning in your stomach. You can consume up to 7 tablets or capsules of hydrochloric acid at one meal. If after consuming the hydrochloric acid or capsules you feel a warmth or burning in your stomach then you have consumed too much hydrochloric acid. It is a good idea to repeat the same dosage at another meal to be sure the warming in the stomach was due to hydrochloric acid and not the food. If you still feel a warmth in your stomach after consuming the same number of hydrochloric acid capsules or tablets then you have taken too much. You should then take one less tablet or capsule at mealtimes to help digest your food. As your stomach regains its ability to produce hydrochloric acid you may then experience a warmth after taking a lower dose. You should then continue to decrease the number of hydrochloric acid tablets or capsules you consume at mealtime. You should notice a marked improvement in digestion and a rapid disappearance of symptoms caused by low stomach acid production.

Hiatus Hernia

The esophagus passes through a small opening in the diaphragm muscle to connect to the stomach. A hiatal hernia occurs when a portion of the stomach bulges through this opening in the diaphragm into the thorax. Hiatal hernias are estimated to occur in 50% of the population over the age of 50 years.

A barium x-ray is the best way to accurately diagnose the occurence of a hiatal hernia. The patient, who has fasted since the previous evening reports to the x-ray laboratory in the morning. A mixture known as a barium meal containing barium sulphate, water and perhaps a flavoring is then swallowed. The barium illuminates the structures on x-ray films. X-rays are then taken of the stomach and perhaps the duodenum and small intestine if necessary. The presence of a hiatal hernia usually shows up on a barium x-ray. Barium x-rays can also be used to diagnose peptic ulcers.

Contrary to proper belief, hiatus hernia does not suddenly appear after the age of 50 years. The development of hiatus hernia takes years, often decades, before it appears. Hiatus hernia is a result of years of abuse to a sensitive stomach. The development of hiatus hernia can be traced back to childhood when it is at this age that we begin our poor eating habits. Children usually have no discipline and frequently put everything in their mouths without consideration of the consequences. The stomach muscle, like any other muscle in the body, can literally go into spasm. Stomach spasms can occur throughout life as a result of bad diet, poor eating habits and poor food combinations. A chronic case of stomach spasms can literally tear a hole in the diaphragm muscle that separates the chest from the abdomen. As a result, a hiatus hernia occurs.

Stomach Ulcers

Stomach ulcers are ulcerations of excavations that can occur in the lining of the stomach. Stomach ulcers occur in 5 to 10% of the population and involve twice as many men as women. The disease is considered to be an illness of young and middle aged adults, but can occur at any age.

The most common symptom of stomach ulcers is upper abdominal pain that may described as burning, gnawing, cramping or aching. The pain may last for several minutes to two hours and may come in waves. The daily pattern of pain is related to the production of hydrochloric acid in the stomach. Pain is usually better in the morning and following a meal, with food in the stomach to buffer the effects of acid. Pain is usually worse before meals and before bedtime. The pain often last for several days then subsides and reoccurs weeks or months later. Other symptoms include nausea, loss of appetite and weight loss. Three major complications of stomach ulcers include bleeding, anemia and perforations. Bleeding may vary from a small amount of hidden blood that occurs over a period of time, to massive hemorrhage requiring immediate treatment. A perforation can occur when an untreated ulcer literally burns itself through the entire stomach wall. This can lead to serious consequences if left untreated. Less than 5% of stomach ulcers are malignant and are associated with the development of stomach cancer.

The cause of ulcer formation is rarely due to excessive production of hydrochloric acid alone. Most cases represent an imbalance between acid, enzymes, mucous and other potentially damaging agents that protect the delicate lining of the stomach. Mucous is produced in large quantities to help prevent the hydrochloric acid and enzymes from digesting through the stomach wall itself. Ulcers are caused when there is a weakening of the mucous membrane and stomach acid is allowed to irritate the stomach wall.

Conventional medical treatment of stomach ulcers focuses on drug therapy to decrease hydrochloric acid production. Losec, Tagamet (cimetidine) and Zantac (ranitidine) are three of the most common drugs routinely prescribed in ulcer therapy. These drugs decrease histamine release at the nerve endings that supply cells of the stomach that produce hydrochloric acid. These drugs markedly decrease hydrochloric acid production. However, decreasing stomach acid is only part of the problem and drug therapy may compromise proper digestion. Common side effects of these drugs include drowsiness, lethargy, dizziness, diarrhea, skin rash and occasionally liver damage.

Stomach and Sinusitis

There is a strong connection between stomach problems and the development of sinus problems. In oriental medicine acupuncture meridians control the flow of chi or energy through the human body. Acupuncture meridians are simply pathways or circuits of chi or energy. There are twelve main acupuncture meridians that represent important organs in the human body. The stomach meridian originates in the face region just below each eye and extends down towards the mouth and around the jaw. The maxillary sinus is located on either side of the nose and beneath the eyes. The stomach meridian passes directly through the maxillary sinuses. Stomach problems can over-activate the stomach meridian and lead to sinus inflammation. Every individual who sufferes from chronic sinusitis involving the maxillary sinus should be evaluated for stomach problems. Alleviating underlying stomach problems frequently helps to cure chronic sinusitis.

Patient Files

Edward B. was a 44 year old construction contractor who came in our office complaining of heartburn, gas, bloating and abdominal pain. A barium swallow test revealed that he had a stomach ulcer. A lifestyle and dietary review revealed that he consumed 4 cups of coffee per day, consumed a fair amount of refined and processed foods and he smoked 1 pack of cigarettes per day. A routine blood test revealed elevated cholesterol, triglycerides and uric acid levels. A food allergy test helped to identify offending foods. We advised him to make some dietary changes and follow the principles of food combining. We recommended that he quit drinking coffee, increase consumption of whole and unprocessed foods, fresh fruits and vegetables and vegetable juices. We prescribed deglycyrrhizinated licorice and other natural supplement extracts to help heal the ulcer. After only two weeks of following our advice he was excited to report that the heartburn and indigestion had disappeared.

June S. was a 55 year old homemaker and part-time sales clerk who came to our office complaining of hiatus hernia and chronic indigestion. A previous barium x-ray and endoscopy confirmed that she had a hiatus hernia and mild inflammation of the stomach lining. June was also slightly overweight and wanted to lose weight. A food allergy test helped to identify aggravating foods. We advised her to avoid milk, dairy, chocolate, alcohol, sugar and spicy foods. We advised her to make some dietary changes and adhere to the simple principles of food combining. We prescribed digestive enzymes and herbal extracts to help heal the inflammed stomach lining. After one month of following our suggestions she reported that her indigestion and stomach discomfort had significantly improved. She noticed that when she didn't follow these principles her indigestion was much worse.

3

The Liver and Gall Bladder

The liver is a large triangular shaped organ located in the upper right area of the abdomen just below the diaphragm. The liver weighs about two to four kilograms and appears dark red in color. The liver is one of the most complex organs in the entire body. The liver is known to have over 500 different and vital functions. Its manifold functions include the storage and filtration of blood, production of bile, storage of vitamins, conversion of sugars into glycogen, breakdown of fats and production of enzymes and proteins. The liver is one of the most resilient organs in the entire body. We can function normally with only 10% of the liver remaining. The liver is one of the most frequently damaged organs in the human body. Chronic use of drugs including alcohol can easily damage liver cells. Fortunately the liver also has an incredible regeneration capacity. The liver replaces itself with entirely new cells every month.

The gall bladder is a small, hollow, pear-shaped organ located directly beneath the liver. The gall bladder is connected to the liver and small intestine by small tubes called ducts. Bile produced in the liver is stored and concentrated in the gall bladder. The gall bladder contracts and expels bile into the small intestine in response to the presence of food in the intestines. Bile aids in the digestion and absorption of fats and other nutrients and helps to eliminate toxins from the body.

The Liver as a Filter

One of the main functions of the liver is to filter the blood. The liver filters out most toxins that circulate in the blood. Every three to four minutes the liver is capable of filtering all four to five liters of blood in the human body. The liver is also the only organ that has a direct blood supply to the intestines. The liver must filter all material that is absorbed in the small and large intestines. The liver must distinguish between useful nutrients that can be utalized by the body and toxic waste material. Like any filter that is not properly maintained the liver can be congested and overloaded with toxic waste material. Improper lifestyle, poor diet and exposure to pollutants in our environment can contribute to the development of a congested liver. If the liver becomes clogged with toxins then the function of the entire organ can become compromised. Any of the 500 different and vital functions of this organ can become affected. As a result the liver doesn't work properly and general ill-health results.

Kupffer Cells

The inner surface of the liver is lined with millions of kupffer cells. Kupffer cells protrude into liver sinuses that are filled flowing blood. Kupffer cells play an important role of the immune system. The main function of kupffer cells is to filter the blood and identify foreign particles. Once foreign particles are identified they are removed from general circulation. Kupffer cells have a high filtration capacity. They rapidly ingest microorganisms and other foreign particles in the blood. These cells can filter and absorb 99% of bacteria and foreign particles in the blood before they reach the rest of the body. The number of kupffer cells lining the sinuses of the liver increases markedly when increased quantities of particulate matter or other debris are present in the blood. Kupffer cells also help to recycle old, worn out red blood cells. Kupffer cells break down red blood cells, recycle iron and produce bilirubin.

Bile

Bile is a clear, yellow, green or orange fluid produced in the liver and is stored and concentrated in the gall bladder. Bile is composed of over 97% water, bile salts, bilirubin, cholesterol, fats, lecithin, sodium, potassium, calcium, chloride and bicarbonate. The most abundant substance in bile is the bile salts, accounting for about half of the total solids in bile. Bile salts and bilirubin are yellow and green colored compounds that are the major end-product of red blood cell and hemoglobin breakdown. These compounds are highly toxic and they dissolve easily in cell walls throughout the body. The liver produces 700 to 1200 milliliters of bile per day. Bile is an alkaline fluid that helps to neutralize the acidic mixture of food from the stomach. Bile also aids in the digestion and absorption of fats. Bile contains most of the toxins that have been filtered by the liver. Bile is used as a vehicle of elimination for the toxins. Dissolved toxins are transported from the liver and gall bladder into the intestines. From the intestines toxins are passed through stool and eliminated from the body. Bile that contains a high concentration of toxins is considered to be toxic bile. Toxic bile that is not eliminated from the body can build up in the liver and gall bladder and accumulate in the body causing multiple problems.

Jaundice

Jaundice is the term used to describe the yellowish discolouration of the skin, white of the eye and other parts of the body due to excess levels of bile circulating in the blood. Jaundice is not a disease by itself, but is usually a sign of underlying liver or gall bladder dysfunction. Any condition that increases the breakdown of red blood cells and hemoglobin can lead to the accumulation of bile in the body. Liver disease can affect the production of bile and lead to jaundice. The presence of a gall stone in the common bile duct can prevent the normal flow of bile from the liver to the intestine. This obstruction can lead a buildup of bile in the body and lead to the development of jaundice.

Gilbert's Syndrome

Gilbert's syndrome is an inherited disorder of bile breakdown that results in elevated levels of bilirubin in the blood. Approximately 2 to 5% of the population have Gilbert's syndrome. This condition is usually benign and asymptomatic, but can occasionally produce mild cases of jaundice. Stress can precipitate high levels of bilirubin.

Sluggish Liver

The term sluggish liver is used to describe a liver that is overloaded with toxins. One of the main functions of the liver is to filter the blood and promote the elimination of toxins. When the liver becomes overloaded with toxins its ability to eliminate these toxins becomes impaired. Toxins build up in the liver and can affect any of the other numerous functions of the liver. The liver literally becomes overburdened and sluggish.

Symptoms of a sluggish liver include fatigue, malaise, lethargy, drowsiness, inability to concentrate, feeling of being drained, depression, unprovoked anger, mood swings headache, indigestion, nausea, gas, bloating, heartburn, stomach aches, nasal congestion, ear congestion, unprovoked allergies, acne, eczema, hives, skin rashes, itchy skin, premenstrual stress, menstrual cramps, menstrual irregularities, muscle aches, muscle weakness, pain and swelling around joints and increased sensitivities to foods and environmental allergens. Signs of a sluggish liver can include right upper abdominal tenderness and yellowish pigmentation to the skin and whites of the eyes.

Conventional diagnosis of a sluggish liver is difficult. Liver function tests are often performed to identify inflammation in this organ. Liver enzymes such as SGOT or AST, SGPT or ALT and GGT usually indicate whether or not there is active inflammation in this organ. Abnormally high levels of these enzymes indicates active inflammation. Active inflammation of the liver is produced when there is only active liver disease. Diseases that can produce active inflammation include cirrhosis, acute hepatitis, chronic hepatitis, acute or chronic biliary tract obstruction and liver cancer. A sluggish liver is not considered an active liver disease. Liver enzymes are usually within normal limits indicating no acute inflammation. Certain non-conventional tests employed by naturopathic physicians can help to identify a sluggish liver.

PMS and a Sluggish Liver

Premenstrual syndrome or PMS is the term used to describe the constellation of symptoms that occur just prior to menstruation in the female menstrual cycle. Symptoms of PMS include behavioral changes, crying, moodiness, irritability, emotional lability, depression, fatigue, increased appetite, acne, breast tenderness, abdominal bloating, abdominal pains, back ache and weight gain. The exact cause of PMS is unknown. However, most researchers now believe there is an imbalance in the female hormones estrogen and progesterone. High levels of estrogen and low levels of progesterone can cause many of the symptoms associated with PMS. The ovaries are directly responsible for producing estrogen and progesterone. However, it is the liver that is ultimately responsible for breaking down and getting rid of these hormones. A sluggish liver that is overloaded and congested can have an impaired ability to breakdown and eliminate these hormones. A sluggish liver can result in hormone imbalances. Treating a sluggish liver should be considered in the treatment of every female with premenstrual syndrome.

Liver Disease

Liver disease is used to describe the group of diseases that affect the liver. Liver disease includes acute and chronic hepatitis, fatty degeneration of the liver, cirrhosis and liver cancer. Hepatitis is an inflammation of the liver characterized by patchy degeneration of liver cells. The major causes of hepatitis are viruses types A, B, non-A non B, alcohol and drugs. Hepatitis A is spread by fecal-oral contact. It causes a "flu-like" illness. Hepatitis B is transmitted through blood and contaminated blood products. Hepatitis B is associated with a wide spectrum of liver disease from an asymptomatic carrier state to acute hepatitis, chronic hepatitis, cirrhosis and liver cancer. Hepatitis B may also cause a "flu-like" illness, but it can progress and ultimately cause liver failure. Chronic hepatitis is an inflammation of the liver that lasts longer than 6 months. Diagnosis of liver disease can be made by a blood test. Elevated liver enzymes including SGOT (AST), SGPT (ALT) and GGT are used to diagnose liver disease.

Fatty Degeneration of the Liver

Accumulation of fat deposits in the liver results in liver degeneration. The liver can store up to forty percent of its weight in fats. Fatty degeneration of the liver is a direct result of poor diet and lifestyle. The most common cause of fatty degeneration is chronic alcoholism. Other causes of fatty degeneration include hepatitis, cirrhosis and liver cancer.

Gall Bladder

The function of the gall bladder is store and concentrate bile from the liver. Although the liver produces over one liter of bile per day the maximum volume of the gall bladder is only 30 to 60 milliliters. Nevertheless, as much as twelve hours of bile secretion can be stored in the gall bladder because water, sodium, chloride and most other minerals are continually absorbed by the gall bladder wall, concentrating the other bile constituents including the bile salts, cholesterol, lecithin and bilirubin. Bile is normally concentrated about fivefold, but it can be concentrated up to a maximum of 12 to 18-fold.

Gall Bladder, Headaches and Sinusitis

There is a strong connection between a toxic gall bladder and the development of headaches and sinusitis. A significant proportion of headaches and sinus inflammation are a direct result of having a toxic gall bladder. In oriental medicine acupuncture meridians control the flow of chi or energy throughout the human body. Meridians are simply pathways of chi or energy. Twelve major meridians are named after the most important organs in the human body. The gall bladder meridian has a unique connection to the top of the face and head. The gall bladder meridian begins directly on the outside of each eye and flows over the forehead over the frontal sinus to the back of the head. If the gall bladder is overloaded with toxic bile then the gall bladder meridian becomes over-activated. An over-activated gall bladder meridian can trigger pain and inflammation anywhere over the length of this meridian. Headaches around the eyes, above the eyes, in the temporal region, over the top of the head and at the base of the skull may be triggered by a toxic gall bladder. This can include all types of headaches including cluster headaches, migraine headaches and tension headaches. The frontal sinuses are located directly above each eye beneath the forehead. The frontal sinuses are located directly in the pathway of the gall bladder meridian. A toxic gall bladder can trigger frontal sinus problems. The unique connection between the gall bladder, headaches and sinusitis should be carefully explored in all individuals with recurrent headaches and chronic sinus problems.

Gallstones

Gallstones are hard, stone-like masses that form in the gall bladder and the duct leading from the gall bladder to the small intestine. Acute inflammation of the gall bladder results in severe pain in the right upper abdominal region, fever, nausea, prostration and occasionally jaundice. Chronic inflammation of the gall bladder results in habitual indigestion accompanied by flatulence and nausea. The indigestion is most evident after a heavy meal or a meal high in fat.

Gallstones affect 20% of all women and 8% of all men over the age of forty years. One million cases of gallstones are diagnosed annually in North America and over 500,000 gall bladder operations are performed each year. Overweight and obese females over the age of forty years are more likely to be affected than men.

Gallstones may be asymptomatic and produce no symptoms at all for many years. Transient colicky pain in the upper right and mid-abdominal areas is usually the first symptom of stone formation. The pain may be dull to excruciating and may last for several hours and may radiate to the back and the right shoulder blade. Nausea, vomiting, fever and chills indicate an acute attack. Stones may block the outlet for the gall bladder and may pass through the duct into the small intestine. If they obstruct the outlet or bile duct then the pain may become excruciating and can lead to jaundice, pancreatitis and infection.

Gallstone formation is the result of many years of a high fat diet, especially high in saturated fats. Obesity and family history are other factors that strongly contribute to the development of gallstones. Additional risk factors include use of estrogen and birth control pills, use of cholesterol reducing medication such as cholestyramine, lovastatin and mevacor, diabetes, liver disease, pancreatic disease and pregnancy.

Diagnosis of gallstones is based on history and location of pain. X-ray and ultrasound usually confirm the presumption of gallstones. Conventional medical treatment of gallstones focuses on surgical operations to remove the inflammed gall bladder. Drugs such Chenodeoxycholic acid or CDCA and Chenodiol are occasionally used to dissolve small stones. It is alarming to note that gall bladder surgeries are performed three times more commonly in North America than in Europe.

Gall Bladder Flush

A gall bladder flush is an old, folk treatment used to help the liver to flush out bile and the gall bladder to contract expelling bile into the small intestine. The flush consists of consuming a mixture that contains equal parts of olive oil with an acid juice such as lemon juice, grapefruit juice or apple cider vinegar. The combination of an unsaturated oil such as olive oil with an acid juice such as lemon juice stimulates the release of bile from the liver and causes the gall bladder to strongly contract expelling its contents into the small intestine. The quantity of mixture consumed depends on the individual's health and their desire for internal cleansing. One or two tablespoons of oil mixed with one or two tablespoons of acid juice is usually sufficient for a mild to moderate flushing of the liver and gall bladder. One or two ounces of oil mixed with one to two ounces of acid juice is sufficient to produce a strong flushing of the liver and gall bladder. The mixture is consumed in the evening before bedtime two hours after a light supper. The next day six to eight glasses of natural lemon juice, grapefruit juice or apple cider vinegar should by consumed. Twelve to forty-eight hours after consumption of the original mixture contents of the liver and gall bladder can be passed in stool. Frequently, yellow and green material will show up in feces. The Gall bladder flush may repeated up to three times. It should be emphasized that the gall bladder flush should be performed on the advice of a licensed health care professional. Contraction of the gall bladder can forcibly expel gallstones in the bile duct and lead to an acute obstruction which can cause excruciating pain and may warrant surgical intervention.

Patient Files

Beth G. was a 33 year old travel agent who came into our office complaining of terrible premenstrual syndrome symptoms. She experienced mood swings, behavioral changes, breast tenderness and backache. She also complained of headaches, indigestion and bloating. She was also slightly overweight and wanted to lose weight. A dietary and lifestyle analysis revealed that she consumed four cups of coffee per day, consumed a diet high in fats and refined carbohydrates and smoked one pack of cigarettes per day. A routine blood test revealed congestion in the liver and gall bladder region. We diagnosed Mary with a sluggish liver. We advised her to make some simple dietary changes and follow the principles of food combining. We recommended that she specifically consume foods that help to promote elimination in the liver. We prescribed natural supplements designed to help clean out her liver and gall bladder. After two months of following our advise she stated that she felt better, did not experience headaches and had no premenstrual discomfort.

Mary C. was a 44 year old waitress who into came to our office complaining of indigestion, gas, bloating and heartburn. Mary was also forty pounds overweight and wanted to go on a diet. Physical examination revealed tenderness in the right upper abdomen area over the gall bladder. We suspected she might have biliary tract or gall bladder obstruction. A routine blood test revealed that she had slight inflammation in the liver and gall bladder region. We advised her to get an abdominal ultrasound. The ultrasound confirmed our suspicions that she had gallstones. A diet analysis revealed that Mary consumed a diet high in fats and refined carbohydrates. We advised Mary to make some simple dietary changes and follow the principles of food combining. We prescribed natural supplements designed to help clean her gall bladder. We advised Mary to try a gallbladder flush. She phoned our office after several days and stated that she had passed many small green, waxy stones in her stool. After two months of following our instructions she stated that she felt much better, her digestion was much improved and she had lost weight.

4

The Pancreas

The pancreas is a large, elongated gland located behind the stomach between the spleen and the duodenum. The pancreas plays two important roles in digestion. It produces a large quantity of digestive enzymes that help to break down and digest food. It also plays an important role in blood sugar regulation. The pancreas produces the hormone insulin that helps to regulate blood sugar levels.

Pancreatic Juice

The pancreas produces important enzymes to help digest carbohydrates, fats and proteins. Pancreatic enzymes breakdown large food particles into small molecules that are easily absorbed across the small intestine into the bloodstream. Pancreatic amylase is an enzyme that digests carbohydrates. Amylase breaks down large complex carbohydrates into simple sugars. Lipase is an enzyme that digests fats. Lipase breaks down large fat molecules into fatty acids and triglycerides. Protease is an enzyme that digests proteins. The stomach produces the hormone pepsin that splits large protein molecules into chunks. Protease enzymes from the pancreas breakdown the protein chunks into small amino acids. The pancreas also produces a large quantity of bicarbonate ions. Bicarbonate neutralizes the acid from the stomach. The collection of pancreatic enzymes, bicarbonate and other fluids is known as pancreatic juice.

Ampulla of Vater

The pancreas connects to the first portion of the small intestine via a small tube or duct called the pancreatic duct. The common bile duct is a small tube that connects the liver and gall bladder to the small intestine. Together the pancreatic duct and the common bile duct attach to each other and connect to the small intestine. The opening in the small intestine is called the ampulla of vater. Pancreatic juice enters into the small intestine through the ampulla of vater. Spasming of the pancreatic duct or the ampulla of vater can prevent pancreatic juice from reaching the small intestine. This can hamper digestion and assimilation of nutrients. The presence of biliary sludge and gallstones are the most common cause of this obstruction.

Enzymes and Indigestion

Pancreatic enzymes are necessary for proper digestion and absorption of nutrients. As long as we eat simple foods and small meals, the pancreas produces enough enzymes to digest food completely. However, when we continually overeat and mix large quantities of rich food the pancreas can become exhausted. An exhausted pancreas does not produce adequate amounts of enzymes to digest foods completely. As a result foods are not completely digested and nutrients are not absorbed.

Stomach and Pancreas

There is a strong connection between the stomach and pancreas. Digestion really begins in the stomach. Digestion in the stomach precedes digestion in the pancreas. The purpose of stomach digestion is to partially breakdown food so that it can be digested by the pancreas. Enzymes in the stomach breakdown food into small chunks that can be more easily digested by the pancreas. Partially digested food then passes into the first portion of the small intestine. Pancreatic enzymes are released into the small intestine to further complete digestion. If the stomach hasn't done its job correctly then this affects the quality of digestion in the small intestine. Poor digestion in the stomach leads to poor digestion from the pancreas.

Islets of Langerhans

Islets of Langerhans are collections of specialized cells located throughout the pancreas. The islets contain three different cells called alpha, beta and delta. Alpha cells produce the hormone glucagon. Glucagon is produced when blood sugar levels are low. Glucagon increases blood sugar levels by increasing sugar release from cells of the body. Beta cells produce the hormone insulin. Delta cells produce the hormone gastrin that stimulates production of digestive enzymes in the stomach.

Insulin

Insulin is a small protein hormone produced in the beta cells of the islets of langerhans in the pancreas. Insulin is the main hormone involved in blood sugar regulation. Insulin is released into the blood when blood sugar levels rise above normal. Insulin promotes the uptake of sugar by cells throughout the body. Insulin also increases the formation of glycogen. Glycogen is a long sugar polymer that is used for sugar storage. Insulin also increases uptake of amino acids, increases protein and fat production and decreases the breakdown of sugar, muscle and fat.

Hypoglycemia

Hypoglycemia is a condition when abnormally low blood sugar levels occur. This condition can result from an excessive rate of removal of sugar from the blood or from decreased release of sugar into the blood. A diet high in sugar and refined carbohydrates leads to a condition known as reactive hypoglycemia. Sugar and refined carbohydrates quickly raise blood sugar levels but later leads to hypoglycemia. Overproduction of insulin from the islets of langerhans leads to an increased rate of removal of sugar from the blood. When a large amount of sugar is consumed this quickly raises blood sugar levels and the pancreas responds by producing a large amount of insulin. Insulin rapidly increases absorption of sugar by body cells. However, the body cells often absorb more sugar from the blood and this results in abnormally low blood sugar levels. A diet high in sugar and refined carbohydrates often leads to a "yo-yo" effect on blood sugar levels.

Diabetes

Diabetes is a medical condition characterized by abnormally elevated blood sugar levels. Diabetes usually involves a problem with the production of the hormone insulin in the pancreas. There are two types of diabetes. Type I or insulin dependent diabetes accounts for about 5 to 10 percent of all diabetics. As its name suggests insulin dependent diabetics require daily insulin shots to help maintain proper blood sugar levels. This condition is usually genetic origin and affects children and young adults. Type II or non-insulin dependent diabetes accounts for 90 to 95 percent of all diabetics. As its name suggests non-insulin dependent diabetics do not require daily insulin shots to maintain proper blood sugar levels. This condition is usually due to a diet high in sugar and refined carbohydrates. The majority of individuals with non-insulin dependent diabetics are overweight and lead a sedentary lifestyle. A diet rich in sugar and refined carbohydrates requires a large amount of insulin to maintain proper blood sugar levels. The repeated demand to metabolize a large amount of simple carbohydrates literally exhausts the beta cells in the pancreas that produce insulin. Treatment of type II diabetes focuses on dietary modification and moderate exercise. With proper diet and exercise the beta cells are able to recharge and are able to supply the body with necessary insulin levels to maintain proper blood sugar levels.

Pancreatitis

Pancreatitis is inflammation of the pancreas. Inflammation occurs when pancreatic enzymes literally digest the pancreas tissue itself. Acute pancreatitis can be caused by many different factors but alcohol abuse is by far the most common cause. Excess use of drugs such as acetaminophen, diuretics and steroids can cause pancreatitis. Mechanical obstruction of the bile tract, usually due to the presence of gallstones is another frequent cause. Chronic pancreatitis usually is a result of chronic irritation to the pancreas. With chronic pancreatitis there is usually digestive dysfunction. There is maldigestion and malabsorption of carbohydrates, fats and proteins. The individual with chronic pancreatitis complains of bulky, fatty, foul smelling stools, weight loss, fatigue, malaise, nausea and vomiting. Poor absorption of vitamins and minerals occurs, particularly calcium and vitamin B12.

Patient Files

Carol R. was a 25 year old law student who came to our office complaining of fatigue, inability to concentrate, dizziness, blurred vision, trembling hands and tingling in her skin. She described herself as a type A personality and her lifestyle as high stress. She also smoked approximately one pack of cigarettes per day. Dietary review revealed that Carol consumed 4 to 5 cups of coffee per day, consumed a diet high in sugar and refined carbohydrates and she frequently ate in fast food restaurants. A routine blood test revealed normal iron levels and low normal blood sugar levels. Carol informed us that her father was diagnosed two years ago with diabetes. We suspected that Carol suffered from hypoglycemia. We advised Carol to make some simple dietary changes and follow with principles of food combining. We recommended that she quit drinking coffee, decrease her sugar consumption and increase consumption of whole foods, grains and vegetables. We suggested that she snack frequently on high protein snacks. We recom-

mended natural supplements to help stabilize her blood sugar levels. After two months of following our advice she informed us that she felt much better, had more energy and was able to think more clearly.

Mike G. was a 54 year old railroad labourer who came to our clinic complaining of indigestion, bloating, flatulence, foul smelling stools. Mike was also overweight and was told by one doctor that he was a borderline diabetic. Five years ago he was also diagnosed with a duodenal ulcer. Dietary review revealed that Mike ate a standard meat and potatoes diet and consumed a large quantity of sugar and refined carbohydrates. A routine blood test revealed moderately elevated blood sugar, high triglyceride and high cholesterol levels. Physical examination revealed upper abdominal tenderness just below the stomach. We advised him to make some dietary changes and follow the principles of food combining. We prescribed pancreatic enzymes and other natural supplements to help improve his digestion and support his pancreas. After three months of following our advice he reported that his digestion had improved considerably and he had lost 15 pounds.

5

The Small Intestine

The small intestine is a long, narrow, hollow tube that is over 6 meters or 20 feet long and connects the stomach to the large intestine. The main purpose of the small intestine is to facilitate complete digestion of food and absorption of nutrients in the blood. The small intestine has three parts; the duodenum, jejunum and the ileum. Partially digested food from the stomach enters the first part of the small intestine called the duodenum. At this site enzymes from the liver, gall bladder and pancreas mix with food and help to digest food. In the jejunum and ileum the digested food particles are absorbed into the blood system.

Duodenum

The duodenum is the first portion of the small intestine that is connected to the stomach. The duodenum is a C-chaped tube about 25 centimeters or 10 inches in length. It plays an important role in digestion because it is where the gall bladder and the pancreas empty their contents. The common bile duct from the gall bladder and the pancreatic duct empty into a small opening called the ampulla of vater. It is at the ampulla of vater that bile and pancreatic enzymes are passed into the duodenum.

Jejunum

The jejunum is the longest portion of the small intestine that extends from the duodenum to the ileum. Most digestion and absorption occurs in this region of the small intestine. The lining of the intestines are thrown into deep folds and minute finger-like projections called villi. The folds and villi increase the surface area of the intestines tremendously. The increased surface area greatly enhances the area available for absorption of nutrients.

Ileum

The ileum is the terminal portion of the small intestine that connects the jejunum to the large intestine. The ileum is also the narrowest portion of the small intestine. All food contain a mixture of different carbohydrates, fats and proteins. These molecules are far too large to be directly absorbed into the blood system. Along the whole length of the jejunum and ileum carbohydrates, fats and proteins are broken down by pancreatic enzymes and bile into simple sugars, fatty acids and amino acids. The simple sugars, fatty acids and amino acids are small enough to pass through the folds and villi of the jejunum and ileum.

Ileocecal Valve

The ileocecal valve is a small one-way valve that separates the small intestine from the large intestine. This valve is located in the right lower abdominal area in the same region where the appendix is located. The purpose of the ileocecal valve is to allow unilateral passage of the unabsorbed contents of the small intestine into the large intestine. The bulky, undigested parts of food passes through the ileocecal valve The ileocecal valve is also an extremely sensitive valve. Too much coarse, scratchy foods can irritate this valve and can result in ileocecal spasming.

Absorption

One of the main purposes of the small intestine is to facilitate absorption of nutrients. An enormous amount of nutrients must pass through the lining of the small intestine into the blood stream. Simple sugars, fatty acids, amino acids, vitamins and minerals must be absorbed through the intestinal wall. To facilitate better absorption the lining of the small intestines is thrown into deep folds and minute projections. These folds and projections are called villi and microvilli. These villi and microvilli tremendously enhance the surface area available to absorb nutrients. The entire surface area of the small intestine is enough to cover the surface of two entire tennis courts. This enlarged surface area makes absorption of nutrients much easier. The lining of the small intestine is very thin. In some areas only one intestinal cell separates the opening of the intestine from a blood vessel. This thin lining enhances ease of transport of nutrients across the intestines.

Nutrients are transported across the intestinal wall in one of three ways. Nutrients can pass through holes or ports between cells of the small intestine. Larger molecules can literally slip through cracks in the lining of the small intestine into the blood stream. Nutrients can pass directly through the intestinal cells themselves. This often requires energy to allow nutrients to pass from the intestinal opening, through an intestinal cell into the bloodstream. Smaller nutrients can pass through the intestine in this way. Nutrients can also pass through the intestines with the help of carrier proteins. Large protein molecules stick out into the opening of the intestines and span the entire distance through the intestinal wall to the bloodstream. Small and medium sized nutrients can pass through the intestinal wall this way. However, this method requires energy to move the nutrients across the intestinal wall. Many nutrients share common transport systems and must compete against each other to be absorbed first. Many amino acids share common transport proteins and must compete against each other to be the first to be absorbed. Many vitamins and minerals also share common transport mechanisms and must compete against each other to be absorbed.

The small intestine has a unique connection to the liver. Once food particles are absorbed into the bloodstream they are carried by the bloodstream directly to the liver. The liver acts as a big filter and food processor. The liver literally filters out good nutrients from bad nutrients. It prepares nutrients for transport throughout the body. It also removes unwanted waste materials and toxins from the system before they enter general circulation.

Malabsorption

Malabsorption occurs when there is impaired absorption of nutrients. Malabsorption is marked by poor absorption of nutrients in the small intestine and results in excessive loss of nutrients in the stool. Malabsorption can result from several different conditions. Three main causes of malabsorption are a defect in the digestive process, an abnormality in the absorptive surface of the small intestine or lymphatic obstruction.

Leaky Gut

A leaky gut is the term used to describe the condition in which large holes in the small intestine occur. Numerous holes in the lining of the small intestine allows for the passage of partially digested food particles into the bloodstream. These food particles wouldn't be absorbed under normal circumstances. They are too large to pass through the normal lining of the small intestine. Their presence along the inner lining of the small intestine and into the bloodstream creates multiple problems. The presence of large, undigested food molecules along the inner lining of the intestine literally clogs up the intestines. This disrupts absorption for all other smaller nutrients that are normally absorbed. As a result, malabsorption and nutritional deficiencies can occur. When large food molecules leak through the gut and pass into general circulation the immune system can become activated. The immune system recognizes normally occuring small molecules, but doesn't normally recognize these large molecules. As a result an allergic reaction can occur. The immune system can manufacture protein molecules called antibodies that selectively seek out and tag these large foreign molecules. Once these large molecules are tagged other immune cells seek them out and destroy them. Leaky gut syndrome has been associated with acne, eczema, psoriasis and other skin problems.

Duodenal Ulcer

A duodenal ulcer is a small ulceration or cavitation of the lining of the duodenum. Like stomach ulcers, duodenal ulcers can cause considerable pain and discomfort. Upper abdominal burning, gnawing, cramping or aching is often described. Pain and discomfort is often worse one to two hours after a meal.

Patient Files

Tami M. was a 34 year old photographer who came to our clinic complaining of eczema, nasal congestion, indigestion, bloating and gas. She often experienced periods of either constipation and diarrhea. Her symptoms were made worse during periods of stress. A routine blood test was normal. A stool analysis was negative for parasites. Dietary analysis revealed a standard american diet high in fats, sugar and refined carbohydrates. She consumed several cups of coffee per day and large amounts of milk. A food sensitivity test revealed multiple allergies. We diagnosed her with leaky gut syndrome. We placed her on a hypo-allergenic diet and advised her to make some simple dietary changes. We recommended several natural supplements to help improve her digestion and to help repair the lining of the small intestine. After two months of following our advice she was happy to report that her eczema was much better. Her nasal congestion had decreased and her digestion was significantly improved.

Jennifer L. was a 30 year old newspaper reporter who came to our clinic complaining of acute abdominal pains, bloating and indigestion. She had previously visited the local hospital emergency room. They originally diagnosed her with possible appendicitis. However, after the doctors reviewed the blood tests and x-rays they ruled out appendicitis. She visited her family physician. He diagnosed her with premenstrual stress. She experienced no relief from her symptoms. She then went to see a gastroenterologist. After performing a barium enema and endoscopy the specialist diagnosed her with irritable bowel syndrome. Unsatisfied she went to a gynecologist for another examination which again proved to be negative. When she came to our clinic she was confused and still experienced the same symptoms. Physical examination revealed tenderness and bloating in the lower abdominal area. There was extreme localized tenderness in the right lower abdominal area near the ileocecal valve. Lifestyle analysis revealed Jennifer was a highly stressful individual. Dietary review revealed a high fiber diet with a lot of raw vegetables and fruit. She was extremely diet oriented and her favorite snack was popcorn. We diagnosed her with irritable bowel syndrome and ileocecal valve spasm. We advised her to make some dietary changes and follow the simple principles of food combining. We recommended that she avoid coarse, scratchy foods. We asked her to avoid a high fiber foods, decrease consumption of salads, raw vegetables and raw fruit. We also asked her to stop eating popcorn. We recommended natural supplements to help relax her intestines and ileocecal valve. After one month of following our recommendations she was delighted to report that her symptoms had improved significantly. She felt better, her digestion had improved and she experienced less pain and bloating.

6

The Colon

The colon or large intestine plays an important role in the digestive process. The colon extends from the part of the small intestine called the ileum to the anus or rectum. The large intestine is approximately 60 inches or 1.5 meters in length and consists of the ascending, transverse, descending, sigmoid colon and rectum. Beginning at the cecum the ascending colon passes upward to the liver and takes a sharp right bend. It continues from this bend as the transverse colon passing below the stomach to the spleen and takes a sharp left bend. After the sharp left bend it takes a downward direction as the descending colon. The descending colon continues to the lower left abdominal area where it forms a S-shaped sigmoid colon. The terminal portion of the colon is known as the rectum.

The function of the large intestine is to absorb water and electrolytes and the store the residual products of digestion. No digestive enzymes are produced in the colon, but an alkaline fluid aids in the completion of digestion begun in the small intestine. Numerous bacteria are found throughout the colon and are capable of digesting and fermenting the indigestible matter in the large intestine. The bacteria are also capable of forming vitamin B1, vitamin B2, vitamin B12, vitamin K and various gases that contribute to flatus in the colon, including carbon dioxide, hydrogen and methane gas. Vitamin K is especially important as the amount of this vitamin in the ingested foods is normally insufficient to maintain adequate blood coagulation.

End-products of Digestion

Feces are the normal end product of digestion and are stored in the colon and rectum. Feces are composed of about three-fourths water and one-fourth solid matter, consisting of about 30% dead bacteria, 10 to 20% fat,

10 to 20% inorganic matter, 2 to 3% protein and 30% undigested roughage of the food and dried constituents of digestive juices.

Peristalsis

Movement of material through the large intestine involves contraction of longitudinal and circular muscles of the colon wall. The wave-like contractions of these muscles is known as peristalsis. These longitudinal and circular muscles are under nervous and hormonal control. Nerves innervate these muscles resulting in propulsion of the digestive material down through the large intestine.

Irritable Bowel Syndrome - Part I

Irritable bowel syndrome is a common, benign disorder of colon or large intestine function. It is typically characterized by episodes of diarrhea, often alternating with episodes of constipation. Irritable bowel syndrome is also known as functional bowel disease, irritable colon, mucous colitis, nervous colitis and spastic colon.

Symptoms of IBS include diarrhea, constipation; often alternating between periods of diarrhea and constipation, abdominal pain, cramping, bloating, flatulence, belching, nausea, vomiting, heartburn, variable appetite, poor digestion and difficult swallowing. Fever, intestinal bleeding and weight loss are not part of the syndrome and usually suggest a more severe underlying disorder. Associated symptoms include emotional lability, depression, anxiety, neuroses, lethargy, headaches and heart palpitations.

The cause of irritable bowel syndrome is not known and no underlying physiological cause has been demonstrated. It is generally agreed that IBS is a disorder of abnormal colon motility. Abnormal colon motility results in altered bowel function and can lead to diarrhea, constipation, nausea, abdominal pain, flatulence and bloating. Factors that affect colon motility include psychological and emotional stressors and diet, especially a diet high in fiber and refined carbohydrates.

There is a strong association between psychological state and irritable bowel syndrome. Particular personality traits have been attributed to the stereotypical individual with IBS. These individuals are typically rigid, methodical persons who are conscientous, borderlining on obsessive-compulsive tendencies. Depression, anxiety, hysteria and neuroses to varying degress are often associated with IBS. Stress can often precipitate attacks of intestinal spasming.

Some researchers feel that irritable bowel syndrome is a learned behavior. Biofeedback studies indicate that we are capable of either increasing or decreasing digestive responses such as stomach acid production and colon motility. Other researchers have advocated that the lack of fiber of the typical western diet may contribute to irritable bowel syndrome. This theory was made from observation that constipation, diverticular disease and IBS are extremely rare in Africans and third world countries where fiber intake is high.

Irritable Bowel Syndrome - Part II

Many individuals with irritable bowel syndrome are advised by their doctors to increase their daily fiber intake. However, too much fiber can actually cause irritable bowel syndrome. Insoluble fiber doesn't dissolve in water and doesn't mix well with digestive juices. Individuals with IBS are often told to increase consumption of wheat bran. However, wheat bran is an insoluble fiber that is difficult to digest. Insoluble fiber tends to be very coarse and scratchy. The coarse, scratchy fiber can irritate the lining of the small intestine resulting in muscle spasms. Muscular spasms can lead to abdominal bloating, distension, gas, pains and many of the other symptoms associated with irritable bowel syndrome.

Too much coarse, sratchy fiber can irritate the ileocecal valve. The ileocecal valve is a muscular, one-way valve that separates the small intestine from the large intestine. The ileocecal valve is located in the lower right abdominal region near the appendix. Too much coarse, sratchy fiber can irritate the ileocecal valve. Muscles around the valve spasm and the valve shuts preventing food to pass from the small intestine into the colon. Ileocecal valve spasm is often misdiagnosed as appendicitis or uterine cramps in women. Symptoms of ileocecal problems include unexplained abdominal pains, gas and bloating.

Individuals with irritable bowel syndrome are advised to limit their intake of coarse, scratchy fibers. Foods classified as coarse and scratchy include raw vegetables, salads, fruits, whole wheat, multi-grain cereals and grains, granola, popcorn and nuts. Too many of these foods can actually aggravate intestinal problems and lead to irritable bowel syndrome. Individuals that eat too many coarse, scratchy vegetables are better advised to eat easy to digest and softer foods.

Diarrhea

Diarrhea is the condition of rapid movement of fecal mattter through the intestines resulting in abnormally frequent evacuations of watery stools. Poor absorption of water, nutrients and minerals occurs. Diarrhea can occur to any one at any age. Acute attacks of diarrhea can last one to two weeks in duration. Chronic diarrhea can last for several months in duration. Foreign travel and drinking contaminated drinking water is a common cause.

Diarrhea may be caused by many different factors including local irritation to the intestines, malabsorption of certain foods, damage to the intestinal wall and emotional disorders such as irritable bowel syndrome. Local irritaion to the intestines can be caused by bacterial or viral infection and chemical agents including a variety of different drugs. Damage to the intestinal wall can be caused by crohn's disease, ulcerative colitis, tuberculosis, lymphoma and cancer. Malabsorption of fats, bile salts, lactose, mannitol, sorbitol and other sugars and carbohydrates can result in diarrhea. Altered intestinal transit time resulting in rapid movement of material can by caused by surgery including small or large intestine resection, stomach surgery and use of certain drugs including the antibiotic tetracycline. Emotional factors such as stress and anxiety can cause increased movement of material through the intestines and increased production of mucous in the colon. Irritable bowel syndrome is one of the most common causes of chronic diarrhea. Other less common causes of diarrhea include pancreatic disease, liver disease, hyperthyroidism, pelvic inflammatory disease, diabetes mellitus, heavy metal toxicity, food allergies, malnutrition, increased consumption of low calorie sweeteners and laxative abuse. Since diarrhea is a symptom and not a disease, further laboratory and diagnostic procedures may be necessary to determine the exact cause of this condition.

Ulcerative Colitis

Ulcerative colitis is a recurrent chronic disease characterized by extensive ulcerations in the large intestine or colon. Symptoms of ulcerative colitis include abdominal pain and profuse blood and mucous stained diarrhea. The cause is unkown but ulcerative colitis shares many of the same characterisitics as regional enteritis or crohn's disease. The disorder is believed to an auto-immune disorder. The disease is often not limited to the colon but can involve other areas including the joints causing migratory arthritis, inflammation of the low back and ankylosing spondylitis.

There is a strong genetic link with the development of ulcerative colitis and there is a much higher incidence of this disease among close relatives. Ulcerative colitis is slightly more prevalent in females than in males and most often appears between the ages of 30 and 60 years.

The individual with ulcerative colitis suffers from attacks of bloody, mucous diarrhea that are usually precipitated by physical or emotional stress. These attacks can last for days, weeks or even months in some severe instances. Some individuals experience relatively few attacks throughout their lifetime while others experience prolonged bouts that can last for years. Frequent and prolonged attacks of ulcerative colitis can predispose the colon to malignant changes that can lead to cancer. Both acute and chronic diarrhea can lead to fluid and electrolyte imbalance and can cause fever, abdominal cramps and weight loss.

Food allergies and sensitivities are often associated with ulcerative colitis. A food allergy or sensitivity test is useful in identifying offending foods and possible triggers in this illness. Individuals with colitis should avoid too many coarse, scratchy fibers which can tend to irritate the lining of the intestines.

Constipation

Constipation is defined as the infrequent, difficult passage of stool. However it may mean different things to different people. To some people it may mean stools that are infrequent, difficult to expel, hard stool, small stool or the sense of incomplete evacuation.

Constipation is believed to affect between 10 to 20% of the North American population. 25 to 50% of the population over the age of 60 years are affected. The frequency of constipation increases with age. Constipation affects males and females equally. Between 250 and 350 million dollars per year are spent on laxatives in North America alone. The widespread use of laxatives indicates how common constipation actually is.

There is a wide variation in the frequency of normal bowel movements. The frequency of bowel movements varies according to individual body make-up, type of intestine, eating habits, physical activity and cultural habits. Normal bowel movements may mean three movements per day for one person and three movements per week for another person. Therefore, by definition an individual that has less than three bowel movements per week is constipated. However, a change in frequency of movements from three per day to three per week may also indicate constipation. Almost always constipation is due to a delay in the transit time within the large intestine or colon.

A wide variety of factors including diet, physical structure, hormonal, metabolic, connective tissue disorders and drugs can affect colon transit time. Evaluation of individuals suffering with chronic constipation must include a consideration of a wide variety of possible causes. Chronic constipation of one month or longer is due to a motility disorder. Factors that decrease movement of material through the colon include advanced age, sedentary lifestyle, low fiber diet, irritable bowel syndrome, hypothyroidism, inflammatory bowel disease, hirschsprung's disease or toxic megacolon, use of constipating drugs such as iron supplements, pain killers and certain antidepressants and local rectal problems such as hemorrhoids, fissure and tumors. Intestinal obstruction can also cause constipation and the use of laxatives can make this condition worse. Continued use of laxatives can lead to chronic constipation. Constipation can also occur during pregnancy.

Chronic constipation can cause uncomfortable symptoms such as nausea, heartburn, indigestion, headache, depression, insomnia, bad breath, diverticulitis, appendicitis, abdominal pain, low back pain, distress to the rectum, flatulence, hemorrhoids, fissures and hernias.

Constipation, Headaches and Skin Problems

There is a strong association between chronic constipation and the development of headaches and skin problems. The colon stores undigested food particles and aids in the elimination of toxins from the body. With constipation, toxin containing stool remains in the large intestine for a longer period of time than normal. The lining of the large intestine is very thin to allow the absorption of water and other useful nutrients back into the bloodstream. However, with constipation, toxins are reabsorbed through the thin lining back into the blood stream. The toxins can circulate in the blood stream and can cause headaches and skin problems. Cleaning the colon is a very important part of the treatment of headaches, skin problems and other chronic diseases.

Diverticulosis

Diverticulosis is a condition in which small, pouch-like herniations form in the muscular wall of the large intestine, usually the sigmoid colon.

Diverticulitis is an inflammation of these small, saccular herniations usually due to accumulation of bacteria and fecal debris.

Diverticulosis is believed to be caused by increased pressure in the large intestine. The muscular wall of the colon is thin and increased pressure may weaken the wall and lead to the formation of small herniations. The herniations usually range in size from 3 millimeters to 3 centimeters in diameter. A low fiber diet is the most common cause of increased intestinal pressure. The standard north american diet is high in refined carbohydrates, protein and fat and is very low in dietary fiber. Fiber is the undigestible portion of plant tissue. It gives food bulk and speeds up intestinal transit time; the time it take food to travel through the digestive system. Fiber is soft, binds water and fills up the colon without exerting much pressure on the intestinal wall. Lack of dietary fiber leads to chronic constipation. Constipation increases the pressure in the large intestine and leads to the formation of herniations or diverticula. Other conditions that can lead to diverticulosis include increased intestinal spasm, irritable bowel syndrome, increased stress, food allergies, especially to milk, cheese and other dairy products and hypothyroidism. Risk factors for the development of diverticulosis include obesity, atherosclerosis, gall baldder disease and hemorrhoids.

Diverticulosis is usually an asymptomatic disease that produces no symptoms. Occasional symptoms associated with this disorder include constipation, abdominal tenderness and occasional rectal bleeding. Diverticulitis may cause intestinal inflammation, lower left abdominal tenderness, flatulence, gas, constipation or diarrhea, rectal bleeding, mucous discharge, fever and increased white blood cell count.

Patient Files

Rachel B. was a 44 year old travel agent who come to our office complaining of diarrhea and ulcerative colitis. She also complained of indigestion, gas, bloating and cold hands and feet. Dietary analysis revealed a high fiber, high carbohydrate and low fat diet. She rarely consumed sugar or refined carbohydrates. She admitted she drank two glasses of milk per day and consumed cheese on a daily basis. Physical examination revealed lower abdominal tenderness with specific tenderness over the sigmoid colon and ileocecal valve. Blood test revealed low normal protein levels, moderately elevated cholesterol levels and low normal thyroid gland function. Food allergy testing helped to reveal many offending foods. We advised Rachel to make some dietary changes and follow the principles of food combining. We recommended she avoid all milk, cheese and dairy products. We prescribed natural supplements to help improve bowel function and help stimulate thyroid gland function. After six weeks of following our advice she reported that she had more energy, she experienced less diarrhea and her colon was functioning much better.

George S. was a 92 year old retired farmer who came to our clinic complaining of chronic constipation. He did not have a regular bowel movement for up to one week. He also complained of fatigue, headaches and poor circulation in his hands and feet. He lived in a local retirement home, did not exercise and lead a sedentary lifestyle. Dietary analysis revealed a high fat, high starch and low fiber diet. He also told us he didn't like vegetables and seldom ate fruit. A routine blood test revealed abnormally low iron levels. A barium enema previously done by his medical doctor revealed multiple diverticula throughout the colon. We advised George to make some dietary changes and follow the principles of food combining. We advised him to increase his fiber intake. We prescribed a psyllium fiber supplement, digestive enzymes and a natural iron supplement. After following our instructions for two weeks he informed us he had daily bowel movements and his energy level was improving.

7

The Immune System

Diseases affecting the system have reached epidemic proportions. AIDS, chronic fatigue syndrome, yeast infection, cancer, allergies and auto-immune disorders including lupus and ulcerative colitis assault the immune system. Never before in the history of mankind have so many different chemicals been circulating in the environment. The immune system is literally bombarded by poisonous chemicals, toxins, pesticides, insecticides, food additives, preservatives and pollutants. Deadly viruses, bacteria and parasites also attack the immune system and render the body incapable of responding to infection. Diseases that affect the immune system and compromise immune function are the plague of the 21st century.

The concept of immune support is a central principle of naturopathic medical practice. Naturopathic physicians have recognized that many different factors are known to affect immune function. Poor diet and improper nutrition, stressful lifestyle, smoking and poor personal hygiene can adversely affect immune function. Specific vitamin, mineral and food supplements are known to stimulate immune function. Specific botanical and herbal preparations have been used for centuries by different cultures to enhance immune function. Exciting new scientific research is being conducted on plant and animal preparations throughout the world and is validating many medicines used in folk medicine. The concept of immune support will undoubtedly become a cornerstone of modern medical practice.

The immune system is a collection of different glands and white blood cells that help the body fight infection and resist disease. The immune system is composed of different glands including the thymus gland, spleen, tonsils, adenoids, lymphatic nodes and the lymphatic system. The immune system is composed of different white blood cells including neutrophils, monocytes, lymphocytes, basophils and eosinophils. Immunity is the ability to resist infection by bacteria, viruses, fungi, parasites and other foreign and toxic substances.

Thymus Gland

The thymus gland is located in the upper chest region just beneath the sternum bone. During late fetal life and the early neonatal period it entraps immature white blood cells called T-lymphocytes or T-cells arising from the bone marrow and circulating in the blood. The thymus processes these cells causing them to become sensitized and capable of developing into the type of white blood cell that is essential to the immune system. After these cells are sensitized they are allowed to re-enter the blood and are transported to lymph tissue where they are stored and wait to be used by the immune system.

If the thymus is removed or becomes non-functional during fetal life then an important part of the body's immunity fails to develop. It is the arm of immunity that is mainly responsible for rejection of organ transplants, natural resistance to cancer and resistance to microbial infection.

The thymus gland produces several hormones including thymosin, thymopoetin and thymic factor. These hormones stimulate thymus gland activity and the development and sensitization of T-cells and regulate their function in the immune system.

The thymus gland reaches its maximum development during puberty and continues to play an important role in the immune system throughout life. After puberty the thymus gland begins to shrink and atrophy as a result of the aging process, stress, radiation, free radical damage, infection, chronic illness and nutritional deficiencies. However, a healthy thymus gland in adults is necessary for a healthy immune system. Nutrients that are specifically required for thymus gland function include vitamin B6, vitamin C and zinc.

While there is no doubt that the thymus plays a major role in the complex immune system, the precise mechanism by which this takes place is not entirely known. As research continues the thymus gland will continue to play an increasingly important role in the immune system and ways in which this mechanism can be manipulated to benefit man will be discovered.

Lymphatic System

The lymphatic system consists of small lymphatic vessels, lymph and lymph nodes. Lymphatic vessels parallel blood vessels and circulate a fluid called lymph. A collection of tissue called lymph nodes are interspersed among the vessels.

The body contains three main types of fluid including blood, lymph and tissue fluid. The fluid portion of the blood excluding red and white blood cells seeps through the capillary walls and circulates among the body tissues. When the fluid is drained from the tissues and is collected by the lymphatic system and it is called lymph.

Lymph is a transparent, usually slightly yellow liquid found within the lymphatic vessels and collected from tissues in all parts of the body and returned to the blood via the lymphatic system. Lymph is about 95% water. The remainder consists of proteins and other chemical substances contained in blood plasma and a specific type of white blood cell called the lymphocyte. Eventually the lymph is collected and dumped back into the bloodstream.

Lymph nodes or glands are accumulations of lymph tissue that are interspersed along the lymphatic system. Lymph nodes are the main source of a specific type of white blood cell called lymphocytes. They also act as an important filter of lymph fluid and remove bacteria, parasites and any foreign or toxic substances. Lymph nodes also play an important role in antibody production.

Spleen

The spleen is a large lymphatic organ located in the upper abdomen on the left side and is just lateral to the end of the stomach. The spleen contains the largest collection of lymph tissue in the entire body. In the normal adult the spleen is about 12.5 to 15.0 centimeters or 5 to 6 inches long and weighs about 2 to 3 kilograms or 5 to 7 pounds. With the presence of disease the spleen enlarges.

The spleen has many important functions. In the unborn child the spleen produces red blood cells. After birth, this function is taken over by the bone marrow. However, the spleen can again produce red blood cells if necessary. In the normal adult the spleen contains a high concentration of red blood cells. In times of exertion, emotional and physical stress, severe bleeding, pregnancy, carbon monoxide poisoning or other occasions when the oxygen in the blood is decreased, the spleen contracts rhythmically to release its stored or red blood cells into circulation. The spleen filters the blood for bacteria, parasites and other foreign or toxic substances. The spleen also produces a chemical called tuftsin. Tuftsin is a small protein that stimulates production of a type of white blood cell called a T-lymphocyte or T-cell.

Liver

The liver is one of the most important organs in the body that has over 500 different functions. The liver is located in the upper right region of the abdomen just beneath the diaphragm. Among its many functions include the storage and filtration of blood, production of bile, breakdown of sugar into energy, the production and breakdown of fats. The liver filters and destroys bacteria and parasites, detoxifies the body from drugs, alcohol and environmental poisons and produces proteins that help to regulate blood volume, build muscle tissue and proteins used in the immune system. The liver also contains millions of cells called kupffer cells that line the liver sinuses. Kupffer cells filter out blood and remove any foreign particles or bacteria from general circulation.

White Blood Cells

White blood cells are the policemen of the immune system. They circulate in the blood and lymph system and seek out and destroy bacteria, viruses, parasites and any other foreign or toxic substances that enter the body.

Neutrophils

Neutrophils are the foot soldiers of the immune system. Their main function is to seek out, engulf and destroy bacteria, parasites and other foreign invaders of the body.

Eosinophils and Basophils

Eosinophils and Basophils play an important role in allergic reactions. Their main function is recognize foreign allergens such as pollen, dust, animal dander, bacterial toxins and release histamine.

Lymphocytes

Lymphocytes are officers of the immune system. There are several different types of lymphocytes that have very different functions. T-lymphocytes or T-cells include T-helper, T-suppressor and killer T-cells. Their function is to either stimulate or suppress immune system function. B-lymphocytes or B-cells produce proteins called antibodies that recognize and stick to the surfaces of bacteria, parasites and other foreign particles. They tag these foreign substances for other cells to attack and destroy. Natural killer cells are lymphocytes that work along side the neutrophils in seeking out, engulfing and destroying foreign invaders.

Monocytes

Monocytes are the garbage collectors of the immune system. After the battle with neutrophils they are responsible for cleaning up the remnants. They engulf and destroy any remaining material.

Macrophages

Macrophages are modified monocytes that take up residence in specific organs of the body. Macrophages are found in the liver, spleen, lungs and lymph system. Like monocytes, they engulf and destroy any bacterial remnants or cellular debris that remains in the body.

Mast Cells

Mast cells are cousins to basophils that play an important role in allergic reactions and are responsible for release of histamine.

Special Chemicals

Special chemicals are produced by the body and exert powerful effects on the immune system. These special chemicals allow the body to communicate with the immune system. The body produces interleukin, complement and interferon and other chemicals. Interleukin is a chemical that activates macrophages and T-cells. Complement is a group of proteins produced in the liver and spleen that work alongside the neutrophils in recognizing and destroying foreign invaders. Interferon is a powerful chemical messenger produced by infected cells in the body.

Interferon is sent to other neighboring healthy cells and warns them of the impending danger of infection.

Stress and Immune Response

Stress can lower immunity and impair the immune response. It is no surprise that most people usually catch colds, flus or other infections when we are under the most stress. Stress impairs all aspects of the immune system. Stress impairs that ability of white blood cells to recognize foreign particles, bacteria, viruses and fungi. Stressors should be identified and reduced. Exercise, rest, sleep, meditation, yoga and biofeedback are excellent ways to reduce stress.

Diet and the Immune System

Diet plays an important role in all aspects of immune function. Sugar and refined carbohydrates can depress immune function. Sugar impairs immune response and directly competes with vitamin C for uptake into white blood cells. Consumption of all fats including saturated, unsaturated and cholesterol should be limited. A high fat diet lowers immunity. Excessive consumption of alcohol can it lower immunity. Consumption of whole and unprocessed foods, fresh fruits and vegetables should be encouraged to optimize immune function.

Patient Files

Sally W. was a 4 year old girl who was brought to our clinic by her distraught mother complaining of frequent colds and flus. Her mother informed us that Sally had at least eight infections in the last year. When Sally was younger she frequently suffered from frequent ear infections. She was always prescribed antibiotics for the infections, which seemed to help somewhat, but another infection would always occur later. Physical examination revealed enlarged, slightly red tonsils. Dietary analysis revealed that Sally consumed a fair amount of milk and dairy products and sugar and refined carbohydrates. We advised her mother to make some dietary changes, decrease milk and dairy consumption and limit the amount of sugar and refined carbohydrates. Food sensitivity testing helped to identify offending foods. We prescribed natural supplements to help build up Sally's immune system. After two months of following our advice her mother reported that Sally had not had an infection.

Carl A. a 62 year old carpenter who came to our clinic complaining of chronic colds and flus. He had been suffering from the last cold for six weeks and just couldn't shake this infection. He was previously prescribed a course of antibiotics which didn't seem to help. Physical examination revealed multiple, tender lymph nodes in the head and neck region and a red, posterior throat. A blood test revealed moderately elevated lymphocytes indicating viral infection. Dietary analysis revealed that Carl consumed a standard american diet high in fats and refined foods. He also consumed 4 to 5 cups of coffee per day and he frequently snacked on sweets. We recommended that Carl make dietary changes to help improve his immune system. We prescribed natural supplements to help stimulate his immune system and help fight viral infection. After three weeks of following our advice he reported that he had finally gotten over that tenacious infection. He also had more energy and he felt significantly better.

8

Hormones and Glands

A hormone is a chemical produced by cells of the body and transported by the bloodstream to the cells and organs on which it has a specific regulatory effect. Hormones act as chemical messengers to body organs stimulating certain life processes and inhibiting others. Hormonal activity is mostly concerned with regulating metabolic activities by controlling the rates at which chemical reactions take place within cells, the transport of substances across cell walls and activities relating to growth and reproduction. The interactions between hormones and metabolic activities throughout the body are controlled by negative feedback. The system is a closed loop in which either an excess or deficit of some hormones initiates a response that results in its return to a level within normal range.

Hormones are produced by various organs and body tissues but are mainly produced by the endocrine glands. The major endocrine glands are the pituitary, pineal, thyroid, parathyroid, thymus, pancreas, adrenal, ovaries and testes.

Pituitary Gland

The pituitary gland is a small, pea-shaped gland located at the base of the brain. It is attached to an important brain structure called the hypothalamus. The hypothalamus plays an important role in the function of the pituitary gland by relaying messages to the rest of the body.

The pituitary gland is the master gland for the entire body. The pituitary gland is divided into two parts. The front part of the pituitary gland called the anterior pituitary. The anterior pituitary produces six important hormones that affect other glands throughout the body. The hormones produced by the anterior pituitary are growth hormone, thyroid stimulating hormone, adrenal gland stimulating hormone, prolactin, follicle stimulating hormone and leutinizing hormone. Most of the hormones produced by the anterior pituitary are regulating hormones that help to control the growth, development and proper functioning of other glands throughout the body. The back part of the pituitary is called the posterior pituitary. The posterior pituitary gland produces two hormones that affect fluid retention in the body and uterine contractions in pregnant females.

A healthy pituitary gland is necessary for proper function of all other glands in the human body. Trauma, stress and toxins, especially heavy metal toxins such as lead and mercury, can affect the function of the pituitary gland. Proper diet and nutrients are necessary for a healthy pituitary gland.

Pineal Gland

The pineal gland is a small, pea-shaped gland at the base of the brain near the pituitary gland. In eastern mythology the pineal gland is thought to function as the third eye of the human body. Scientific research now reveals that the pineal gland acts as a sensitive light receptor. The pineal gland produces the hormone melatonin. Melatonin helps to regulate the biological clock within the human body. Production of melatonin helps to affect human behavior within a twenty-four hour time period. It determines both the time to fall sleep, the duration of sleep, time to wake up and the duration we are remain awake. Chronic sleep disturbances, chronic insomnia and seasonal affective disorder are believed to occur as a result abnormalities in melatonin production.

Thyroid Gland

The thyroid gland is the largest of the endocrine glands located in front and on the sides of the neck just below the adam's apple. The thyroid gland produces hormones that are vital for maintaining normal growth and metabolism. This gland is also the largest source of iodine in the human body.

The main hormone produced in the thyroid gland is thyroxine. Thyroxine is made in this gland from a combination of the amino acid, tyrosine and the inorganic mineral, iodine. Thyroxine travels to all cells of the human body and influences the rate of metabolism and growth. Metabolism is the sum of all the physical and chemical processes that occur within the human body. Metabolism is concerned building up and maintaining the body. These processes are concerned with the breakdown of large molecules into small molecules with the release of energy that is supplied to the body.

The rate of metabolism can be increases or decreased by the thyroid gland. The amount of thyroxine produced in the thyroid gland can affect the rate of metabolism like a thermostat affects the temperature setting in the house. The rate of metabolism can also be increased by exercise, by elevated body temperature as with fever which can more than double the metabolic rate, by hormonal activity as with adrenaline and insulin which can both raise the metabolic rate.

Basal Body Temperature

Basal body temperature is the temperature of your body at rest before you have begun to move around or exercise. The normal oral human body temperature ranges between 36.4 to 37.6 degrees celcius or 97.6 to 99.2 degrees fahrenheit. Low oral body temperature below 36.6 degrees celcius or 97.6 degrees fahrenheit suggests low thyroid function. High oral body temperature above 37.6 degrees celcius or 99.2 degrees fahrenheit suggests high thyroid function.

Thyroid Gland Self-Test

Basal Body temperature is a reliable indicator of thyroid gland function. Your basal body temperature is best taken first thing in the morning before you have gotten out of bed. Place an oral themometer on your night stand before you go to bed the previous evening. When you wake up in the morning insert the themometer in your mouth for five minutes before you get out of bed. Record your oral temperature. Repeat this exercise for at least one week. There will be slight variations in daily temperature, but your average temperature over the week should give you an accurate reading how your thyroid gland is functioning.

Hypothyroidism

Hypothyroidism is a deficiency of thyroid gland function and is marked by an underproduction of the hormone, thyroxine. Hypothyroidism occurs in approximately 10 to 15% of the adult population. Mild to severe hypothyroidism occurs in 10 to 12% of the population, while moderate to severe hypothyroidism occurs in 1 to 4% of the population. Hypothyroidism occurs slightly more in females than in males. Hypothyroidism that occurs in children results in delayed physical growth and decreased mental development.

Symptoms of hypothyroidism include physical and mental sluggishness, fatigue, malaise, moderate weight gain, obesity, cold intolerance, cold hands and feet, decreased sexual desire, slowed digestion and constipation. Other symptoms include swelling and edema throughout the body, enlargement of the tongue, brittle, cracked fingernails and dry, thin hair that falls out easily. With females symptoms include menstrual cycle irregularity, an abnormally short or long cycle, prolonged menstruation, infertility, premature birth and miscarriages. With men symptoms include impotence and baldness. High cholesterol and triglycerides, low body temperature, enlarged heart, high blood pressure, impaired kidney function, anemia and delayed tendon reflexes can also occur.

The exact cause of hypothyroidism is unknown. A decrease in thyroid function is a normal part of aging. Heredity seems to play an important role in its development and hypothyroidism occurs more commonly when other family members suffer with the same affliction. Also pituitary gland disorders, radioactive iodine therapy, thyroid surgery, congenital enzyme deficiency, nerve damage and nutritional deficiencies including vitamin A, vitamin E, iodine, zinc and the amino acid, tyrosine can cause low thyroid function. Excessive use of stimulant drugs and diet pills can lower thyroid gland function.

Sluggish Thyroid

Sluggish thyroid is the term used to describe the syndrome that occurs when an individual experiences many of the symptoms of low thyroid function but has normal blood thyroxine levels. Many individuals fall into this dubious category. They experience fatigue, malaise, lethargy, cold intolerance, cold hands and feet, constipation, hair loss and other symptoms of hypothyroidism. However, the blood levels of thyroxine are usually at low normal levels. Eventhough the thyroid produces normal amounts of thyroxine, its effect on the body is blunted. Ultimately it is the effect of thyroxine on the cell's of the body that determines the state of metabolism. Treatment of a sluggish thyroid should focus on nutritional support for the thyroid gland and eliminating any blockages that may inhibit its function in the body.

Parathyroid Gland

The parathyroid glands help to maintain proper calcium balance within the body. The parathyroid glands include a group of four small pea-shaped glands located just beneath the thyroid gland in the neck region. These glands produce parathyroid hormone or PTH which affects blood calcium levels. Low levels of calcium in the blood stimulates the release of parathyroid hormone while high levels of calcium inhibits its release. Parathyroid hormone helps to maintain proper blood calcium levels. It does this by exerting its effects on bone, kidney and the digestive system. In bone it enhances reabsorption of calcium by stimulating the break-down of bone. This affects the release of calcium from bone into the bloodstream. In the kidney, parathyroid hormone increases the elimination of phosphate and increases the reabsorption of calcium. In the digestive system, parathyroid hormone increases the absorption of calcium from the intestines.

Thymus Gland

The thymus gland is the control center for the growth and development of the immune system. The thymus gland is located in the upper chest region beneath the sternum near the heart. The thymus gland produces several hormones including thymosin, thymopoetin and thymic factor. These hormones stimulate thymus gland activity and the development and regulation of an important part of the immune system. The thymus gland plays an important role in the maturation and development of T-lymphocytes or T-cells. A healthy thyroid gland is necessary for a healthy immune system.

Adrenal Glands

The adrenal glands are a pair of triangular glands located at the top of the kidneys and they weigh about 5 grams each. The main function of the adrenal glands is to help the body respond to stress. The adrenal glands are divided into an inner area, the medulla, which accounts for 1/5 the size of the gland and on outer area, the cortex, which accounts for 4/5 the size of the gland. The two structures are quite different in their anatomy and the hormones they produce.

The inner medulla produces adrenaline, also called epinephrine and noradrenaline or norepinephrine. These hormones enter the bloodstream and are transported throughout the body where they act as stimulants to the various organs. Adrenaline increases heart rate, increases blood pressure, constricts blood vessels, dilates the bronchi in the lungs, increases metabolic rate and increases muscle activity in the digestive system.

The outer cortex produces more than thirty different types of steroid hormones. There are three major types of hormones produced here depending on their actions. They include aldosterone, sexual hormones and cortisone.

The adrenal cortex produces hormones that maintain proper fluid and electrolyte balance in the blood. The main hormone concerned with fluid and electrolyte balance is aldosterone. Aldosterone maintains proper sodium and chloride minerals in the blood by stimulating their reabsorption from urine in the kidneys. They have the same effect to a lesser degree on the sweat and salivary glands and on the intestines. Additionally, aldosterone promotes the loss of potassium in the urine. The net result of these hormones is maintenance of mineral and electrolyte balance in the blood and the body.

The adrenal cortex produces small amounts of male and female sex hormones. Small quantities of testosterone and estrogen are produced here that have effects throughout the body. The sex hormones are responsible for the secondary sexual characteristics such as the development of facial hair and the deepening of the voice in males and the development of breasts in females.

Another group of hormones produced in the adrenal cortex are concerned with increasing blood sugar levels and supplying sugar to the muscles for energy in the event of an emergency. The main hormone of this group is cortisol or cortisone, which is responsible for 95% of this group's activity. Cortisol increases blood sugar levels. Cortisol promotes the breakdown of carbohydrates, proteins and fats. It increases the formation of glucose in the liver, decreases sugar utilization by the body, increases the breakdown of amino acids and fats into sugars. Cortisol is also a potent anti-inflammatory. Its synthetic derivatives such as cortisone and hydrocortisone are widely used in medicine to reduce inflammation throughout the body. Cortisol is produced in the adrenal glands at a rate of fifteen to twenty milligrams per day under non-stressful conditions. During stress periods this rate is rapidly increased to meet demands placed upon the body. Highest levels of cortisol occur between 6 and 8 AM in the morning, while the lowest levels occur between 10 and 12 PM at night. The production of cortisol is increased during periods of illness, pregnancy and stress.

Adrenal Glands and the Stress Response

The adrenal glands are the main organs in the human body that help you deal with stress. During stressful circumstances the adrenal glands produce small quantities of adrenaline and cortisol. These hormones are directly responsible for the physiological changes that occur in the body. Your heartbeat increases, breathing become shallow and rapid, adrenaline and cortisol are released into the bloodstream, the liver releases stored glucose, your pupils dilate, muscles tense for movement, blood flow decreases to the digestive system, blood flow decreases to the extremities, blood flow increases to the brain and major muscles and the body begins to perspire to cool itself.

Sluggish Adrenal Glands

Sluggish adrenal glands is the term used to describe the syndrome that occurs when the adrenal glands have become overworked and exhausted. The main function of the adrenal glands is to help the body respond to stress. A certain amount of stress is necessary and healthy for the human body. However, an excess amount of stress can literally exhaust the adrenal glands. During each stressful circumstance the adrenal glands pump out a small quantity of adrenaline, cortisol and other hormones. In our modern, secular society the amount and duration of stressful circumstances has increased tremendously. Life, marriage, relationships, finances, travel, work, pollution, crime, war and other stressors are rampant. Constant stress can deplete the adrenal glands and have an adverse effect on health. Individuals with exhausted adrenal glands have an inability to cope with stress. They often experience fatigue, lethargy, malaise, headaches, mood swings, emotional instability, depression, frequent infection, chest pains, heart palpitations, muscle aches, skin rashes, indigestion, heartburn, irritable bowel sydrome, bladder problems, abnormal menstrual periods, infertility, impotence, poor sex drive and chronic yeast infection. Treatment of sluggish adrenal glands focuses at building up and supporting the adrenal glands and eliminating any blockages that may inhibit its function in the body.

Ovaries

The ovaries are a pair of almond-shaped glands located in the lower abdomen on either side of the uterus in females. The ovaries have two basic functions: the production of eggs and the production of female hormones. The ovaries produce fertile eggs that are released from the ovaries each month. The ovaries also produce the female hormones estrogen and progesterone. Estrogen and progesterone are responsible for women's feminine physical characteristics and the female reproductive process. The function of the ovaries is connected to the pituitary gland. The pituitary gland produces hormones that travel to the ovaries and influence the production of eggs and hormones. Disruption of the pituitary-ovary connection can affect the normal female reproductive cycle. Treatment of ovarian and reproductive problems should be focused at building up and supporting these glands and eliminating any blockages that could adversely affect the normal female reproductive cycle.

Testes

The testes are a pair of egg-shaped glands located on the exterior of the lower abdomen. The testes have two basic functions: the production of sperm and the production of male hormones. The testes produce fertile sperm that can be united with the female ovum and lead to conception. The testes also produce the male hormone testosterone. Testosterone is responsible for the male's masculine physical characteristics and the male reproductive process. The function of the testes is connected to the pituitary gland. The pituitary gland produces hormones that travel to the testes and influence the production of sperm and hormones. Disruption of the pituitary-testes connection can affect the normal male reproductive cycle. Treatment of the testes and reproductive problems should be focused at building up and supporting these glands and eliminating any blockages that could adversely affect the normal male reproductive cycle.

Patient Files

Audrey D. was a 43 year old medical secretary who came to our office complaining of fatigue, depression, indigestion, constipation and an irregular menstrual cycle. She also complained of cold hands and feet and hair loss. Dietary analysis revealed a relatively healthy diet consisting of whole foods, fresh fruits and vegetables. She did not drink coffee, consume an excessive amount of sugar or refined carbohydrates or consume an excessive amount of processed foods. A routine blood test revealed low normal thyroid hormone levels. We instructed Audrey to take her body temperature first thing in the morning before getting out of bed for two weeks. Her body temperature revealed an abnormally low basal body temperature. We diagnosed Audrey with a a sluggish thyroid.

We advised her to make some dietary changes and follow the principles of food combining. We prescribed natural supplements to help get her thyroid gland working better. After two months of following our recommendations Audrey informed us that she felt much better, had more energy and her hands and feet were warmer.

Dan M. was a 30 year old teacher who came to our office complaining of fatigue, depression, muscle weakness, stress and inability to cope with day to day activities. He also complained about indigestion and heartburn. He informed us that he was under a lot of stress. He had just started a new teaching job, his wife was pregnant and he was experiencing financial difficulties. Dietary analysis revealed that he drank three to four cups of coffee per day, consumed a moderate amount of sugar and refined carbohydrates and consumed alcohol on a day to day basis. Physical examination revealed small, tight pupils and a considerable amount of stress rings in the eyes. His blood pressure dropped a significant amount when he changed position from a supine position to a standing position. We diagnosed Dan with sluggish, overworked adrenal glands. We advised Dan to make dietary changes and follow the simple priniciples of food combining. We prescribed natural supplements to help support and build up his adrenal glands. After one month of following our recommendations he informed us that he felt much better, his energy and his depression had significantly improved.

PART II

Foods, Disease and Health

9

Caffeine

Caffeine is one of the most popular and widely used and drugs in North America. Caffeine is also one of the most abused and addictive drugs. Caffeine is widely available in coffee, tea, chocolate and in a variety of over-the-counter medicines in the pharmacy. Coffee is the drug of choice for millions who regularly consume the beverage in the morning or throughout the day. Tea toddlers who consume teas regularly consume equal amounts of caffeine.

Problems associated with excess caffeine consumption include angina, anxiety, attention deficit disorder, bedwetting, behavioral changes, bladder cancer, bladder irritation, breast tenderness, depression, diabetes, diarrhea, fatigue, fibrocystic breast disease, heart disease, heartburn, heart papitations, high blood cholesterol, high blood pressure, hyperactivity, hypoglycemia, inability to concentrate, indigestion, insomnia, irritability, irritable bowel syndrome, mood changes, muscle spasms, nightmares, osteoporosis, panic attacks, peptic ulcers, peri-anal itching, poor sleep, possible birth defects during pregnancy, premenstrual stress, prostatitis, rectal burning, restlessness, restless leg syndrome, ringing in the ear, stomach cancer, stomach irritation, tremors in hands and extremities, trouble swallowing and urinary tract infections.

A Personal Testimonial

I can still remember being a student at college and university. I would start my morning with one or two big cups of coffee to help me wake up and attend those dreaded early morning classes. Between classes I would sit in the cafeteria and consume several more cups of coffee. In the afternoon I would have another cup to help me stay awake in those boring afternoon classes. In the evening I have a cup of tea to help me stay awake and study late at night. This cycle was repeated each semester.

Then I decided to attend naturopathic medical college in Seattle, Washington. My coffee consumption continued. It was there that I was introduced to gourmet coffee including flavoured coffee, expresso and cafe latte. Every morning on my way to naturopathic medical college I would stop at the 7-11 and get a big cup of coffee to go. I knew I had a problem during second year of medical college when I was in a morning nutrition class. There I was sitting in the back of the room drinking my big cup of coffee and listening to the teacher lecture on the bad and evil effects of caffeine. I knew I had to quit. The teacher challenged me to quit for two weeks. I accepted the challenge and suffered the effects of caffeine withdrawal for one week. Unfortunately I resumed my coffee consumption with the approach of mid-term exams. However, I did quit coffee completely the day after I graduated from naturopathic medical school. I no longer wake up and search the house for coffee to start my day like a half-starved lunatic.

What Is Caffeine?

Caffeine is a small nitrogen containing chemical that belongs to a group of drugs called methylxanthines. It is found naturally in coffee, green and black tea, cocoa and chocolate and several other plants. It is also added to a variety of over-the-counter medicines for pain relief, anti-sleep and weight loss products. Caffeine is also widely used in most "natural" and "herbal" products used to increase energy, delay fatigue, increase endurance and promote weight loss.

Physiological Effects of Caffeine

Caffeine is a central nervous system stimulant. In low to moderate doses caffeine can cause mild cortical arousal with increased alertness and deferral of fatigue. It can also cause behavioral changes, restlessness, nervousness, insomnia, anxiety, ringing in the ears, muscular tremor and lightheadness. In sensitive individuals even a few sips of coffee can cause nervousness and insomnia. Very high doses of caffeine can cause respiratory problems and convulsions.

Caffeine and Metabolism

Caffeine is a metabolic stimulant. It can increase blood fat levels, increase and decrease blood sugar levels, lead to dehydration and deplete the body of minerals and water soluble vitamins. There is also some evidence that large doses of caffeine over long periods of time can cause pancreatic cancer.

Caffeine and the Heart

Caffeine can increase the heart rate, increase blood pressure, induce heart palpitations, decrease blood flow to the brain and decrease blood flow to the extremities causing cold hands and feet.

Caffeine and the Digestive System

Caffeine can stimulate hydrochloric acid production in the stomach, increase enzyme production from the pancreas and increase muscle contractions throughout the digestive system. It can also cause indigestion, heartburn, nausea, vomiting, stomach irritation, peptic ulcers, intestinal spasms, diarrhea and anal itching. It is important to note that caffeine is not the only substance in coffee and tea that can cause these effects on the digestive system. Decaffeinated beverages can just as easily irritate the digestive system.

Caffeine and the Kidneys

Caffeine is a diuretic on the kidneys and the urinary tract. It can increase both the frequency and quantity of urination. It can cause kidney and bladder irritation, burning and itching sensation with urination.

Caffeine and the Sweat Glands

Caffeine can increase activity and sweating in sweat glands throughout the body. Caffeine can also stimulate activity in modified sweat glands in breast tissue in females. Excess caffeine consumption is associated with fibrocystic breast development.

Caffeine and Immune Function

Caffeine can decrease immune function, decrease thymus gland size and decrease levels of circulating antibodies. Excess caffeine consumption can impair the ability of the immune system to respond to infection.

Caffeine and Muscles

Caffeine can cause smooth muscle relaxation, especially to the bronchi which can increase the air supply to the lungs. This makes caffeine useful in treating asthma. It can also improve contraction of the diaphragm in individuals with chronic obstructive lung diseases. Caffeine can also stimulate skeletal muscle contraction and delay muscle fatigue throughout the body.

Caffeine and Pregnancy

Caffeine in low to moderate doses is generally regarded as safe during pregnancy. The safety of high doses of caffeine exposure to the developing fetus is still unknown. Caffeine is known to cross the placenta and passes unchanged through breast milk. It can then cause all the above physiological effects on the fetus as it does to the mother who consumes it. Caffeine consumption by the mother can contribute to nervous irritability, insomnia and colic in infants.

Beneficial Effects of Caffeine

Not all effects of caffeine are bad. There are many beneficial effects of caffeine. Caffeine is widely used to increase brain activity, prevent fatigue, increase endurance, delay the onset of sleep, acts as a mild decongestant with allergies, helps improve air supply in asthmatics and in individuals with chronic obstructive lung disease.

Decaffeinated beverages

Decaffeinated coffee and tea beverages are often used as substitute for the real thing. They look and taste like the original beverage but have only trace amounts of caffeine.

The original decaffeination process involved steaming the coffee beans or tea leaves in water for 24 to 48 hours. A liquid solvent was then percolated through the substance. The solvent was able to remove up to 97% of the caffeine content. The solvent extraction would then be repeated if necessary to remove additional caffeine. The chemicals used as solvents include acetone, benzene, chloroform, ethanol, ethyl acetate, ethyl ether, formaldehyde, methylene chloride and trichlorethylene. After the solvent extraction procedure residual amounts of the chemicals would remain in the original substance. Some of the solvents including benzene, chloroform and trichlorethylene are suspected and known carcinogens which can cause cancer.

In first year college chemistry laboratory we extracted caffeine from super-saturated black tea. The process was relatively simple and after we evaporated the solution we were left with a teaspoon of white powder called caffeine.

The two most popular solvents used today are ethyl acetate and methylene chloride. A water-only decaffeination process was developed in Switzerland in 1979. This novel process only involved water as the solvent. The water-only decaffeination products tend to be slightly higher in price than the regularly decaffeinated products.

It is important to note that decaffeinated beverages also contain other chemicals which can have deleterious effects on the human body. Tannins and resins from coffee and tea can irritate the stomach and digestive system and can irritate the skin. Residual amounts of solvents used in the decaffeination process can irritate the body.

Caffeine Content of Common Beverages and Foods

Item	Milligrams Caffeine
Brewed drip coffee (6 ounces)	100-180
Brewed percolated coffee (6 ounces)	90-170
Instant coffee (6 ounces)	60-120
Decaffeinated brewed coffee (6 ounces)	2-5
Decaffeinated instant coffee (6 ounces)	1-5
Tea - North American variety (6 ounces)	40-100
Tea - Imported variety (6 ounces)	40-120
Instant tea (6 ounces)	30-60
Iced Tea (12 ounces)	60-80
Hot Chocolate (6 ounces)	5-25
Chocolate milk (8 ounces)	3-8
Milk Chocolate (1 ounce)	2-20
Dark Chocolate (1 ounce)	5-40
Baker's Chocolate (1 ounce)	20-30
Chocolate flavored syrup (1 ounce)	2-5
Mountain Dew (12 ounces)	54
Coca-Cola (12 ounces)	45.6

Diet Coke (12 ounces)	45.6
Dr. Pepper (12 ounces)	39.6
Pepsi-Cola (12 ounces)	38.4
Diet Pepsi (12 ounces)	36.0
Canada Dry Ginger Ale (12 ounces)	32.0
Canada Dr Diet Cola (12 ounces)	1.2
NoDoz (per tablet)	100
Vivarin (per tablet)	200
Anacin - Maximum Strength (per tablet)	32
Excedrin (per tablet)	65
Midol (per tablet)	32
Aqua Ban (per tablet)	100
Cafegot (per tablet)	100
Fiorinal (per tablet)	40
Darvon (per tablet)	32

Patient Files

Bill W. was a 45 year old middle management executive at Costco. He came in complaining of fatigue, lethargy and insomnia. He also experienced occasional heart palpitations. After questioning Bill about his lifestyle and dietary habits he stated that he consumed 20 to 30 cups of coffee per day. He usually ate breakfast on the run consisting of several cups of coffee and donuts. He consumed copious amounts of coffee throughout the day. He frequently ate lunch at fast food restaurants and ate a standard dinner of meat and potatoes. He also smoked 1 pack of cigarettes per day. We calculated Bill's total caffeine intake as 3000 to 4500 mg per day. We advised Bill to make some simple dietary changes including decreasing his coffee intake to 5 cups per day. Abstaining from his usual amounts of coffee was very hard at first. He experienced normal withdrawal symptoms of moodiness, irritability and headaches. However, after 1 month he was consuming no coffee whatsoever. His energy level had improved significantly, he was eating better and he had no trouble sleeping.

Alice M. was a 33 year old accountant and competitive squash player who came in our clinic complaining of facial acne and premenstrual tension. PMS symptoms included moodiness, irritability, breast tenderness, sugar cravings, abdominal bloating, swelling and fluid retention. She also experienced back ache and terrible cramps with menstruation. She stated she wanted to lose some weight. After questioning her about dietary habits she stated she consumed 5 to 10 cups of coffee per day. We advised her to make some simple dietary changes including quitting coffee for at least 3 months. Her facial acne improved, her PMS disappeared, she lost some weight and her squash game improved. She stated the single most important factor that contributed to her health was quitting caffeine intake.

10

Fats and Oils

Fats and oils are an important part of the diet. However, a high fat diet is associated with degenerative disease including heart disease, stroke, auto-immune diseases and cancer. There are different types of fats and it is important to realize that not all fats are created equal. There are good and bad fats and oils. Good fats and oils are beneficial and help to support body processes. Bad fats are harmful and have negative effects on the body. It is important to realize the differences between various fats and oils so that you can make wise dietary choices.

Problems with high fat intake include abdominal bloating, acne, allergies, angina, arthritis, atherosclerosis, autoimmune disorders, breast cancer, cardiovascular disease, chest pain, colon cancer, constipation, diabetes, dizziness, fatigue, gall bladder disease, gallstones, gout, hearing loss, heart disease, high blood pressure, high blood cholesterol, high blood triglycerides, impotence, indigestion, kidney disease, kidney stones, menstrual difficulties, menstrual cramps, obesity, overweight, peripheral vascular disease, premenstrual syndrome, senility, skin rashes, stroke, transient ischemic attacks or TIA's and vertigo.

Functions of Fat

Fats have very important functions in the body. Fats are a normal constituent of cell walls in all tissues of body. Strong cell membranes helps to keep bacteria, viruses and other foreign substances from entering the body. They are used to make hormones, vitamin D, and bile in the liver. They are also used to make prostaglandins, important hormone-like substances that have strong effects throughout the body. Fats are a necessary and vital requirement of the human body and must be consumed from the diet. However, excess consumption of fat and oils may have harmful effects on the human body.

Excess Fat Consumption

The main problem with fats is that we consume too much of them. Fats contain twice as many calories as either carbohydrates or protein. One gram of fat produces 9 calories of energy. One gram of carbohydrate or protein produces only 4 calories of energy. High fat foods include fast foods, junk foods, fried foods, desserts, milk, cheese and other dairy products and red meat. The average North American consumers 40 to 50% of their total caloric intake as fats. This amount is too high. A more desirable fat intake would be 10 to 20% of total caloric intake.

Fats and Oils

The main difference between fats and oils is that fats are solid at room temperature and oils are liquid at room temperature. Animal products including chicken, beef, pork, lamb, turkey and fish contain fats. Vegetable oils including safflower, sunflower, corn, olive and flaxseed oil are oils. Foods generally contain a mixture of different fats, although one type of fat or oil usually predominates. They are three different types of fats; saturated, mono-unsaturated and poly-unsaturated fats.

Saturated Fats

Saturated fats are solid at room temperature and as their name suggests they are saturated with hydrogen atoms. Animal sources include chicken, beef, pork, lamb, organ meats, milk, cheese, butter, ice cream and other dairy products. Vegetable sources include coconut, cocoa butter, palm oil, palm-kernel oil, commercially baked goods, pie filling, non-dairy substitutes and fast food preparations. Saturated fats are very stable and resistant to heat, light and chemical change. They inhibit the production of good prostaglandins and form prostaglandins that are not beneficial to the body. Saturated fat is also closely aligned with cholesterol and is associated with heart disease, stroke, cancer and other diseases. The main problem with saturated fats is that we eat too much of them.

Mono-unsaturated Fats

Mono-unsaturated fats are liquid at room temperature. Sources of mono-unsaturated oils include olive, avocado, peanut and canola oils. Olive oil is probable the highest source of these type of fats.

Poly-unsaturated Fats

Poly-unsaturated fats or PUFA's are liquid at room temperature and as their name suggests they are not full with hydrogen atoms. Animal sources include mother's milk, organ meats, salmon, halibut, cod, tuna, sardines, herring, trout and other fish. Vegetable sources include linseed, flax, soy bean, walnut, corn, sunflower, sesame, cotton seed and oil of most green leafy vegetables.

Fat Content of Common Beverages and Foods

Item	Grams Fat
Water - fresh tapwater (1 cup)	0
Apple - with the skin (1 medium)	0
Grapefruit (1 medium)	0
Orange (1 medium)	0
Pear (1 medium)	0
Avocado (1 medium)	20-30
Beets (1 medium)	0
Cabbage (1/2 cup)	0
Broccoli (1/2 cup)	0-1
Brussel Sprouts (1/2 cup)	0-1
Potato (1 medium)	0-1
Spinach (1/2 cup)	0
Bread - white flour (1 slice)	1-2
Bread - whole wheat flour (1 slice)	1-2
Bread - with garlic butter(1 slice)	9-12
Cream of Wheat (1/2 cup)	0-2
Oatmeal (1/2 cup)	0-1
Corn Flakes (1/2 cup)	0
Rice Krispies (1/2 cup)	0
Shredded Wheat (1/2 cup)	0
Spaghetti - Regular (2 ounces)	1-3
Almonds (1 ounce)	14-18
Peanuts (1 ounce)	12-16
Peanut Butter - Regular (2 tbsp)	15-18
Pecans (1 ounce)	18-22
Walnuts (1 ounce)	17-20
Butter (1 teaspoon)	4-5
Butter (1 restaurant pat)	4-5
Margarine (1 teaspoon)	4-5

Cheese - Blue (1 ounce)	9-10
Cheese - Cheddar (1 ounce)	8-10
Cheese - Feta (1 ounce)	6-8
Cheese - Mozzarella (1 ounce)	5-10
Cheese - Parmesan (1 ounce)	9-11
Mayonnaise - Real (1 tbsp)	10-12
Chocolate - Semi-sweet chocolate chips (1 ounce)	10-16
Chocolate - Hershey Milk Chocolate (1 ounce)	7-8
Bacon - fried (3 strips)	3-15
Bologna - Beef (1 slice)	7-8
Ham - (1 slice)	3-6
Beef - regular ground (3 ounces)	15-25
Chicken - breast meat without the skin (3 ounces)	3-6
Chicken - breast meat with the skin (3 ounces)	5-9
Pork - regular ground (3 ounces)	15-25
Salmon - fresh (3 ounces)	10-15

Free Radicals and Trans Fats and Oils

Although poly-unsaturated fats and oils are beneficial to the body, two detrimental processes occur to them that make them harmful to the human body.

Free radicals are highly reactive molecules that can be produced by the body or by the environment. They are a normal product of oxidation and are produced by light, heat and as an end product of biochemical reactions within cells. Free radicals target poly-unsaturated fats in the body. They attach themselves to fats in cell membranes and cause degeneration and decay of the cell wall. Free radicals are believed to contribute to heart disease, cancer and premature aging. Antioxidants are natural substances that bind to free radicals and prevent them from attacking cell walls. Vitamin A, beta-carotene, vitamin C, vitamin E and selenium are important nutritional antioxidants. To prevent free radical damage to vegetables oils, place the contents of one or two vitamin E capsules in the bottle of oil.

Trans fats and oils are produced from light, heat and chemical reactions that alter the shape or configuration of the original fat or oil. Trans fats are produced during heating of oils and deep frying of foods. These oils are still used in cell membrane structure and are metabolized to make energy. However, they cannot be used to make prostaglandins and they do not retain essential fatty acid activity. To prevent the formation of trans fats and oils store vegetable oils in cool places or the refrigerator. Avoid all trans fats and oils. Avoid commercially processed oils, margarine and fried foods.

Most vegetable oils on grocery shelves are heated to approximately 120 degrees celcius during commercial processing. Heating leads to the generation of trans fatty acids. Avoid heating oils as in frying. This can also lead to the production of trans fats. Cook with mono-unsaturated oils such as virgin olive oil. To prevent free radical damage and the production or trans fats and oils avoid leaving oils out in sunlight and cook with mono-unsaturated oils.

Commercial Oil Making Process

The process of commercial oil making involves heating the raw, unrefined oil to 120 degrees celcius, expeller pressing under high pressure and heat, solvent extract with hexane and benzene solvents, degumming and the removal of gums and lecithin, bleaching and deodorization with caustic sodas. During this process naturally occuring vitamins and minerals are removed and lost. Synthetic anti-oxidants such as butylated hydroxytoluene or BHT and butylated hydroxyanisole or BHA are added to the processed oils. Heat destroys essential fatty acid activity of the oil and is destroyed during this process.

Cold Pressed Oils

Cold pressed oils are oils are natural and unrefined oils that are processed with the lowest possible temperature. Fifty degrees celcius is the highest temperature that is applied to oil during this process. No external heat above this temperature is applied to the seed while it is being pressed. Cold pressed oils still retain their original, naturally occuring vitamins and minerals and their essential fatty acid activity.

Hydrogenation

Hydrogenation is the process in which hydrogen gas is bubbled through vegetable oils, as in the production of margarine. This process is relatively cheap and the product is a substance that looks and tastes like butter. During this process naturally occuring vitamins and minerals are depleted. Also during this process large amounts of trans fats are produced. These fats are still used to produce energy and are used in cell walls, but they are devoid of essential fat activity. Butter is a naturally produced product that contains its original vitamins and minerals and does not contain high amounts of trans fats. Butter is recommended over margarine.

Toxic Fats and Oils

Toxic fats are oils that contain harmful substances. Canola oil from rape seed and mustard seed contain erucic acid. High levels of erucic acid can cause fatty degeneration of the liver, kidneys, heart and adrenal glands. Oil from cotton seed may contain gossypol. High levels of gossypol can cause indigestion, stomach irritation, shortness of breath and lung problems. Do not consume toxic fats and oils.

Cholesterol

Cholesterol is a hard, yellow, waxy substance that is solid at room temperature. It is a steroid molecule found in animal fats and oils, bile, blood, brain tissue, milk, egg yolk, cheese, fat sheaths around nerves, liver, kidney and adrenal glands. It has many important functions in the body including being an important component of cell membranes, insulation of nerves, brain and other vital organs and is used to make vitamin D in the skin. It is used to make steroid hormones in the ovaries, testes, adrenal glands, kidney and liver including estrogen, progesterone, testosterone and cortisone. It is also used to help make bile in the liver which helps to digest and absorb dietary fats. The body can normally make cholesterol to supplies its daily needs. However, the more cholesterol we eat, the less our body needs to make. A diet high in fats, especially saturated fats and white sugar and refined carbohydrates supplies more cholesterol than the body needs. The average consumption of cholesterol in the diet is 800 milligrams per day. One egg, 1/4 ounce butter and 1/4 ounce of meat has the equivalent of 250 milligrams of cholesterol. Increased levels of cholesterol have been associated with jaundice, liver dysfunction, hypothyroidism, kidney dysfunction, diabetes and cardiovascular disease.

Cholesterol and Atherosclerosis

The role that cholesterol plays in the formation of atherosclerotic plaques in arteries has been the subject of dispute for several decades. Elevated levels of total cholesterol have been associated with heart disease, heart attack and stroke. Cholesterol is found in deposits in arteries with other saturated fats, protein and calcium. These plaques block blood flow through the vessel, narrow the arterial opening and harden the blood vessel. When the artery is sufficiently blocked blood flow is decreased and parts of the body are deprived of vital oxygen and nutrients. Further research has drawn a distinction between different types of cholesterol in the body. Both types are involved in fat transport in the body and include high density lipoprotein or HDL cholesterol and low density lipoprotein or LDL cholesterol. It is now believed that the balance between HDL and LDL is more significant than the total concentration of cholesterol in the blood. The risk of heart disease increases as LDL increases and HDL decreases.

HDL and LDL Cholesterol

HDL promotes the removal of excess cholesterol from the body including the arteries. Its removal from the body is thought to be beneficial rather than harmful. In contrast, LDL picks up cholesterol from ingested fats and from cells that make it in the body and delivers it to blood vessels and muscles where is is deposited in the cells. The concentration of cholesterol in the cells within the linings of the arteries contributes to a buildup of atherosclerotic plaques.

The question of whether or not the dietary intake of fats affects the pattern of HDL and LDL cholesterol levels has not yet been answered to everybody's satisfaction. All experts do agree, however, that those persons who are at high risk for heart disease, have a heart condition or are overweight, should drastically limit the amounts of fats and cholesterol in the foods the eat.

Triglycerides

Triglycerides are compounds that consist of three fatty acids bound with one molecule of glycerol. They are usually a storage fat in animals. They function to insulate the body and conserve heat, surround and protect the body and internal organs and act as a reserve for energy. Excess sugars in the diet are converted to triglycerides for storage. They serve as a fuel for all organs in the body except the brain and can be broken down into sugar again and metabolized for energy. High blood triglycerides are produced from overeating and a diet high in sugar and refined carbohydrates. Elevated blood levels are considered as important as high cholesterol in the development of heart disease, stroke, cancer and other diseases. Tiglycerides make the blood more viscous and sticky and promotes the development of atherosclerosis.

Essential Fats and Oils

It is impossible to live a long and healthy life without some fat in your diet. Certain fats and oils are necessary for proper body function. These specific fats and oils that are required by body are called essential fats and oils. Like vitamins and minerals, the body cannot manufacture them and they are needed in small amounts for proper function. They must be obtained from the diet. Essential fats and oils have important functions in the body. They are involved in creating strong cell walls and membranes, fat metabolism, transport of other substances, antioxidants and prostaglandin production.

There are two main types of essential fats and oils. Omega-3 fats or linolenic fats or LNA and omega-6 fats or linoleic fats or LA. Deficiency of omega-3 oils or LNA can produce growth retardation, muscle weakness, visual impairment, learning disabilities, muscle incoordination, tingling in the arms and legs and behavioral disturbances. Deficiency of omega-6 oils or LA can produce skin rash, eczema, hair loss, dry eyes and mouth, arthritis, circulatory problems, heart disease, decreased immunity, increased infections, decreased wound healing, sterility in males, infertility and miscarriages in females, behavioral disturbances, liver dysfunction and kidney dysfunction. Examples of omega-3 oils or LNA include flaxseed, linseed, hemp seed, whale, salmon, cod liver, catfish, mackarel and other fish and the oil of green leafy vegetables. Flaxseed oil contains approximately 60% of omega-3 oils. These oils contain linolenic acid, eicosapentanoic acid and docosahexanoic acid. Examples of omega-6 or LA include safflower, sunflower, corn, cottonseed, peanut, walnut, soybean, pumpkin, evening primrose and borage. Saffower and evening primrose oils contain the richest source of omega-6 oils. The daily requirement of essential oils is 1 to 3% of total daily caloric intake or 3 to 6 grams per day. Approximately 10% of body fat is composed of essential oils. Vegetarians may contain up to 25% of body fat being composed of essential oils.

Prostaglandins

Fats located in the cell membrane are used to make prostaglandins. They were initially isolated in the prostate gland of men but are now found throughout the human body. Prostaglandins are short lived but powerful hormone-like chemicals that exert strong effects throughout the body. Prostaglandins are derived from poly-unsaturated fats in the body.

They are over 30 different types of prostaglandins that have different effects on the body. Some prostaglandins are derived from essential fats and oils. Essential oils are used to make prostaglandins of the type 1 and 3 series. These prostaglandins have beneficial effects on the human body. They inhibit platelet aggregation, dilate blood vessels and prevent the formation of cholesterol plaques in arteries. They also stimulate the immune system, increase insulin sensitivity and help to balance blood sugar levels, decrease arthritis and joint pain and decrease inflammation. Prostaglandins of the type 1 series are derived from omega-6 oils and prostaglandins of the type 3 series are derived from omega-3 oils. Prostaglandins of the type 2 series are derived from animal fats and have negative effects on the body. They promote platelet aggregation, constrict blood vessels and encourage the formation of cholesterol deposits in arteries. Manipulation of dietary fats and oils can alter the balance between different prostaglandins in favor of prostaglandins of the type 1 and 3 series.

Diet and Fats

Recommended total fat intake should be between 10 and 25% of total caloric intake. Consumption of high fat foods should be decreased. Butter, margarine, milk, cheese and other dairy products, eggs, beef, pork, lamb, chicken, desserts, candy, pastries, peanuts, walnuts, cashews and other nuts, vegetable oils and shortening are high fat foods and their consumption should be limited. Decrease consumption of white sugar, chocolate and refined carbohydrates. Limit consumption of alcohol. Avoid processed and refined foods. Increase consumption of whole and unprocessed foods, fresh fruits and vegetables.

Patient Files

Mary W. was a 55 year old homemaker who into our clinic complaining of high cholesterol, cold hands and feet and ringing in the ears. She was also overweight and wanted to lose weight. After performing a routine blood test we determined her total cholesterol and triglyceride levels were too high. Blood sugar, uric acid and thyroid hormone levels were all within normal limits. After reviewing her diet and lifestyle habits we determined that Mary's fat intake was too high. We placed her on a diet to restrict total fat intake to 20% of total caloric intake. Within 3 months her total cholesterol level dropped significantly. She started a daily exercise program consisting of a 45 minute walk. The circulation to her hands and feet improved and ringing in her ears decreased. She had more energy and she felt much better.

Katherine B. was a 25 year old actress and part-time waitress who complained about fatigue, hair loss, dry skin and brittle nails. Upon questioning she also stated that her menstrual period was irregular and her last menstrual period was about 3 months ago. She was a lacto-ovo vegetarian and consumed no animal products including milk and eggs. After reviewing a one week diet diary we determined her total fat intake was too low. We concluded that she was deficient in essential fats and oils. We recommended that she start to use fats and oils in her daily diet. She was prescribed daily evening primrose oil and sublingual vitamin B12 drops. Within one month the quality of her skin, hair and nails improved significantly. She was more energetic and was no longer fatigued. She was now experiencing a menstrual period approximately once per month.

Mike P. was a 64 year old retired logger who complained of high blood pressure and angina pains in the chest. He was taking blood pressure pills and nitroglycerin tablets to treat his chest pains. After performing a routine blood test we determined that his total cholesterol was high, HDL or "good" cholesterol was too low and LDL or "bad" cholesterol was too high. Triglycerides and uric acid were also elevated. After reviewing his diet and lifestyle habits we determined that Mike consumed too much fat. We calculated his fat intake to be 45% of total caloric intake. We advised Mike to make some simple dietary changes and limit fat intake to 20% of total caloric intake. Within one month after implementing these changes he started to feel better. After 3 months his cholesterol levels improved, his blood pressure decreased significantly and he experienced less chest pain.

11

Fiber

Plant fiber is the portion of plant foods that is not digested in the human digestive system. Fiber is not broken down by digestive enzymes and juices and therefore, passes through the small and large intestines undigested. It it is composed of cellulose, which is the "skeleton" of plants, hemi-celluloses, lignin, pectin, gums mucilages, algae seaweeds and other carbohydrates undigestible in humans.

Problems associated with poor fiber intake include anal fissures, appendicitis, atherosclerosis, autoimmune disorders, colon cancer, colon polyps, constipation, diabetes, diarrhea, diverticulitis, diverticulosis, gallstones, heart disease, hemorrhoids, hiatal hernia, high blood fats, high blood pressure, hypoglycemia, intestinal cancer, irritable bowel syndrome, malabsorption problems, obesity, peptic ulcers, pernicious anemia, rectal cancer, spastic colon, tooth decay, ulcerative colitis and varicose veins

Natural Sources of Fiber

Vegetables, cereals and fruits are the main source of dietary fiber. Although wheat bran is advertised as an excellent source of fiber, it is not unique nor is it as nutritious as fruits and vegetables and some other whole unprocessed cereals. The typical diet in western countries contains 10 to 20 grams of fiber per day. In some rural African communities the typical daily fiber intake is 130 grams per day. A more beneficial and attainable daily fiber intake would be 40 to 60 grams per day. Forty-five percent of daily fiber intake comes from vegetables, 35% from cereals, grains and legumes and 20% from fruits. Meat, chicken, fish, milk, cheese and dairy do not contain fiber.

Cellulose

Cellulose is the best known and most widely distributed component of plant cell walls. It is not water soluble, but is capable of binding water in the gut. Up to 50% of cellulose is digested by bacteria in the colon into short chain fatty acids. The primary effects of cellulose is to increase the bulk of the stool and increase transit time; the time it takes food to pass from the stomach until it is excreted as fecal matter. Vegetables, whole grains and cereals contain large amounts of cellulose. The best known cellulose fiber is wheat bran.

Hemi-cellulose

Hemi-cellulose is also a component of plant cell walls. It is composed of sugar molecules including glucose, mannose, xylose and galactose. It is not water soluble, but is capable of binding water in the gut. Vegetables, whole grains and cereals contains large amounts of hemi-cellulose. The best known hemi-cellulose is oat bran.

Lignin

Lignin is a type of fiber derived from alcohol compounds. It is water soluble and is not digested or absorbed in the colon. It is capable of binding bile salts and other organic compounds in the digestive system. A large amount of lignin in the diet may delay or impair the absorption of some vitamins and minerals. Lignin has demonstrated antibacterial, antiviral, antifungal and anti-cancer effects. Lignin is found in the woody parts of plants, wheat, cereals, apples and cabbage.

Gums

Gums are the sticky material extruded at the site of injury to plants. They are composed of complex sugars called polysaccharides, that form gels. They are water soluble. Gums are used as emulsifiers, thickeners and stabilizers in foods, bulk laxatives and adhesives. Different types of gums include arabic, acacia and karaya gums.

Mucilages

Mucilages are found in the inner portion of plants seeds and are found in most beans and legumes. They are water soluble and are capable of binding large amounts of water. Mucilages are used as thickeners, stabilizers and fiber forming agents in the food industry. They are used in cheese making, salad dressings, ice creams, soup and toothpaste. They are used in the pharmaceutical industry in jellies, lotions, skin creams and laxatives. They are also used to manufacture tobacco and explosives. Different types of mucilages include galactomannan, guar gum and psyllium seed. Galactomannan is derived from the indian custer bean. Glucomannan is derived from konjac root and has been safely consumed for thousands of years in the Orient. The fiber of psyllium seed is capable of binding 30 times its weight in water.

Algae Seaweeds

Algae seaweeds include agar, alginic acid and carrageenan. Agar is used as a bulk laxative and is capable of binding heavy metals in the digestive system. Carageenan is toxic in large doses and can cause stomach ulcerations, liver damage and inflammation throughout the intestines.

High Fiber Foods

Most fiber rich foods contain a mixture of cellulose, hemi-cellulose, lignin, gums, mucilages and algae seaweeds. It is difficult to assign the health benefits a fiber rich food to a specific fiber type since most foods represent a combination of different fibers.

Fiber Content of Common Beverages and Foods

Item	Grams Fiber
Water - fresh tap water (1 cup)	0
Apple - with the skin (1 medium)	3.3
Banana (1 medium)	3.2
Grapefruit (1 medium)	3.2
Orange (1 medium)	2.6
Peach - with the skin (1 medium)	1.8
Pear - with the skin (1 medium)	3.1
Prunes - with the skin (3 medium)	3.0
Apple Juice (1 cup)	0.8
Grape Juice (1 cup)	0.8
Orange Juice (1 cup)	0.8

Broccoli (1/2 cup)	2.2
Cabbage (1/2 cup)	1.4
Cauliflower (1/2 cup)	1.1
Carrots (1/2 cup)	2.3
Celery (1/2 cup)	1.1
Cucumber (1/2 cup)	0.4
Lettuce (1/2 cup)	0.9
Onion (1/2 cup)	0.8
Potato - baked with the skin (1 medium)	3.0
Tomato (1 medium)	1.2
Spinach (1/2 cup)	1.2
Beans - baked (1/2 cup)	8.8
Kidney Beans - cooked (1/2 cup)	7.3
Navy Beans - cooked (1/2 cup)	6.0
Lentils - cooked (1/2 cup)	3.7
Bran Muffin (1 medium)	3.2
Popcorn (3 cups)	1.2
Peanuts (10 nuts)	1.4
All Bran Cereal (1/3 cup)	9.0
Cheerios (1 cup)	1.0
Corn Flakes (1 cup)	1.2
Raisin Bran (1 cup)	4.4
Rice Krispies (1 cup)	0.1
Sugar Smacks (1 cup)	0.5
White Bread Toast (1 slice)	0.6
Whole Wheat Toast (1 slice)	2.1
Spaghetti - regular (1 cup)	1.1
Rice - Brown (1 cup)	1.0
Rice - White, Polished (1 cup)	0.2
Milk 1% (1 cup)	0
Milk 2% (1 cup)	0
Cheese - Cheddar (1 slice)	0
Egg - boiled (1 medium)	0
Beef (3 ounces)	0
Chicken (3 ounces)	0
Pork (3 ounces)	0
Fish (3 ounces)	0

Beneficial Effects of Fiber

Fiber helps to increase stool bulk and increase intestinal transit time, absorbs water, absorbs organic wastes and toxins, stabilizes blood sugar levels, lowers cholesterol and triglycerides and helps to maintain the normal bacterial flora of the intestines. Fiber is effective in treating constipation, diarrhea, diabetes and obesity.

Increased Stool Bulk and Increased Transit Time

The primary effects of dietary fiber are to increase the bulk of the stool and make it softer by taking up water as it passes through the colon. Water insoluble fibers especially cellulose and hemi-cellulose found in wheat bran, increases fecal bulk. Water soluble fibers such as lignins, pectins, gums and mucilages are beneficial in delaying emptying of stomach contents into the small intestine. These fibers increase transit time due to increased gel absorption and has a small effect on fecal bulk. These effects are illustrated in comparing African villages eating a high fiber diet and English men eating a low fiber diet. Intestinal transit time in African villagers was 36 hours compared to 71 hours in English men. Daily fecal output averaged 470 grams for the Africans, while the value for English men averaged 108 grams.

Water Absorption

Water soluble fibers including lignins, pectins, gums, mucilages and storage polysaccharides are water soluble. These fibers have a strong affinity for water and are capable of forming gels. This increases transit time through the digestive system and increases fecal water content. This property is beneficial in treating both constipation and diarrhea.

Absorption of Minerals

Fiber binds minerals including calcium, magnesium, iron and zinc. Fiber can also bind heavy metals such as lead, mercury, arsenic and aluminum. However, this may prevent adequate absorption of trace minerals and lead to electrolyte imbalance in the body.

Absorption of Organic Wastes and Toxins

Fiber is capable of absorbing organic wastes and toxins and carries them out of the intestinal tract. The increase in stool bulk hastens the passage of feces and may reduce the length of time the intestinal wall is exposed to toxins. Fiber absorbs bile salts that are excreted from the liver and gall bladder. Bile transports fat soluble organic compounds and toxins. Fiber is capable of binding cancer causing chemicals that might otherwise pass through the digestive system and be absorbed into the blood system. Fiber is also capable of binding bacterial toxins that are produced in the intestines and prevents them from being absorbed into the body.

Stablization of Blood Sugar Levels

Fiber helps to stabilize blood sugar levels. A high fiber diet increases the bulk of food ingested and delays emptying of stomach contents into the small intestine. This helps to increase release of digestive enzymes and insulin from the pancreas. Sugar release from food is decreased and sustained over a longer period of time. Blood sugar abnormalities are prevented and normal glucose levels are maintained.

Fiber, Cholesterol and Triglycerides

Fiber helps to lower blood cholesterol and triglycerides. Water soluble fibers including lignins, pectins, gums and mucilages are capable of binding cholesterol and triglycerides in the small intestine and prevent their absorption. Water insoluble fibers including cellulose and some hemi-celluloses such as wheat bran, have little effect on reducing blood cholesterol levels. Oat bran is effective in reducing blood cholesterol levels. Cholesterol production in the liver is also reduced due to the binding of bile salts in the intestines. Bile salts are a rich source of cholesterol and are capable of combining with fiber and being excreted through the digestive system. This prevents cholesterol from being absorbed into the blood and increases production and excretion of cholesterol in bile.

Bacterial Flora of the Digestive System

A high fiber diet helps to normalize the bacterial flora of the colon. Fiber is utalized as a food source for good bacteria such as Lactobacillus acidophilus and other related species. Fiber is capable of binding bacterial toxins and excreting them through the stool, thereby preventing their absorption and adverse effects on the human body. Intestinal pH is decreased and an acidic environment helps to prevent overgrowth of unhealthy bacteria.

Short Chain Fatty Acids

Most fibers, except some lignins, are partially digested and fermented in the colon by intestinal bacteria. Pectins and similar water soluble fibers are almost completely digested by these bacteria. By-products of this digestion include water, methane gas and short chain fatty acids. Short chain fatty acids including butyric acid are the prefered source of energy for cells that line the intestinal wall. Some short chain fatty acids are absorbed and transported to the liver where they are broken down to make energy. Other short chain fatty acids help to prevent cancer.

Constipation and Diarrhea

Fiber is beneficial in treating both constipation and diarrhea. A high fiber diet increases stool bulk and decreases transit time through the digestive system, which is beneficial in treating constipation. The gel forming properties of water soluble fibers helps to increase the absorption of water from the intestines. Also the ability of fiber to bind organic substances and toxins helps to prevent diarrhea and aid in elimination.

Obesity

Fiber is important in preventing weight gain and obesity. High fiber foods are high in bulk, low in calories and should be consumed in large quantities. A lot of chewing is required to break down high fiber foods and increased digestive juices, hormones and enzymes are required to digest these foods. A meal high in fiber increases satiety or the sense of fullness and decreases feelings of hunger.

Diabetes

Fiber is important in the treatment of diabetes, hypoglycemia and other blood sugar abnormalities. A high fiber diet delays emptying of stomach contents into the small intestine. A slow and sustained release of foods from the stomach decreases insulin response in the pancreas. A slow release of insulin prevents rapid blood sugar changes in the body. Blood sugar level and glucose response are stabilized and abnormalities in blood sugar levels are prevented. A high fiber diet is also beneficial in helping to control weight problems in diabetics.

Fiber and Diet

A high fiber diet is strongly recommended. Increase consumption of whole and unprocessed grains and cereals, fresh fruits and vegetables. At least 20 to 40 grams of dietary fiber per day is strongly recommended. Fiber can be included in the diet as a daily supplement.

Patient Files

Danielle Z. was an 9 year old child who presented with her mother at our clinic one day. The mother appeared distraught. She stated that Danielle hadn't had a bowel movement in three weeks. She had previously went to the emergency room at the local hospital and the doctor there determined there was no immediate medical emergency. The doctor advised the mother to give her daughter an enema or a laxative. We performed a physical examination which was unremarkable. After reviewing her dietary habits we determined that Danielle's diet was deficient in dietary fiber. She consumed large amounts of sugar and refined carbohydrates, ate fast foods and drank large amounts of soda pop. We advised that Danielle start to increase her dietary fiber intake in the form of vegetables, fruits and whole grains. We also prescribed a daily fiber supplement. After consuming the fiber supplement for three days she started to have regular daily bowel movements.

Max F. was a 72 year old retired railroad worker who suffered from chronic constipation for several years. Bowel movements were often hard and painful. He often resorted to laxatives to help move his bowels. After questioning Max about his dietary habits we determined that he was deficient in dietary fiber. He seldom drank water and consumed a diet rich in refined and processed foods. We advised Max to drink at least 6 to 8 glasses of water per day, increase consumption of dietary fiber in the form of fresh vegetables, fruits and whole grains. We also prescribed a daily fiber supplement. He now experiences regular bowel movements.

12

Milk

Milk was once touted as the perfect food supplying the body with ample amounts of carbohydrates, fats and proteins. We are often reminded by dairy consumer groups that we should drink milk daily to be healthy and to get our daily calcium requirements. However, we should be aware that we are the only species on the earth that continues to consume milk after we are weaned. Cow's milk is certainly good for calves, but is no good for children and is even worse for adults.

Problems associated with milk consumption include acne, allergies, anemia, angina, anorexia or poor appetite, arthritis, asthma, atherosclerosis, attention deficit disorder, bedwetting, behavioral problems, bloating, blood in stools, bronchitis, canker sores, celiac disease, colic, colitis, crohn's disease, depression, diabetes, diarrhea, ear infections, eczema, excess phlegm and mucous, fatigue, flatulence, headaches, heart attack, heartburn, hyperactivity, indigestion, insomnia, irritable bowel syndrome, irritability, kidney problems, lou gehrig's disease, mucous colitis, multiple sclerosis, muscle aches, nasal congestion, nausea, peptic ulcers, post-nasal drip, proteinuria, sinusitis, spastic colon, recurrent strep throat, recurrent tonsillitis, stomach aches, ulcerative colitis and vomiting.

Lactose

Lactose is the primary sugar derived from milk. Lactose is actually two sugars stuck together by a simple chemical bond. The enzyme lactase helps to break this bond and releases two simple sugars, glucose and galactose. Lactase is located in the wall of the small intestine. Lactase breaks down lactose into simple sugars that are then easily absorbed by the body and utalized for energy.

Lactose Intolerance

A hereditary deficiency of lactase occurs in approximately 70 to 90% of asians, 70 to 80% of arabs, 50 to 70% of africans, 50 to 70% of indians, 10 to 20% of scandinavians and 10 to 15% of caucasians. The inability to digest lactose in milk is called lactose intolerance. Lactose intolerance usually manifests itself between infancy and early adulthood. Symptoms of lactose intolerance include abdominal pains, bloating, cramping, diarrhea, flatulence, gas and stomach aches. Many of these symptoms are created by bacteria in the gut that are able to digest and breakdown lactose. During the breakdown process the sugars are fermented and the bacteria release large amounts of gas that results in many of the symptoms associated with lactose intolerance.

One cup of whole milk contains 12.0 grams or 30% of lactose by weight. One cup of 2% milk contains 13.0 grams or 41% of lactose by weight, one cup of skim milk contains 11.4 grams or 57% of lactose by weight. One cup of lowfat yogurt contains 16.0 grams of lactose or 46% lactose by weight. Two ounces of cheddar cheese contains 1.0 gram of lactose or 2% lactose by weight. Cheeses are generally better tolerated by many lactose intolerant individuals, but they are very high in fats and salt and still produce a lot of phlegm and mucous in the body.

Milk Protein

Milk contains over sixty different proteins and over 35 of these proteins have been documented to cause allergic reactions in humans. Two highly allergic proteins in milk are casein and lactalbumin.

Approximately 50% of the protein in milk is from casein. Casein is a rather large protein molecule that is primarily used to make curds and cheese. It was once believed that casein was too large a molecule to be directly absorbed from the intestines and had to be digested first by enzymes in the gut. Current research suggests that considerable amounts of casein are directly absorbed from the intestines and bypass digestion altogether. Once in circulation intact casein molecules combine with large sugar molecules to form slimy complex molecules that increase mucous in the body. Milk is considered a very mucous forming food that literally plugs up various parts of the body. Excess milk consumption is directly related to an excess quantity of phlegm and mucous in the body. Excess phlegm and mucous in the body is related to several diseases including recurrent nasal congestion, post nasal drip, colds, recurrent ear infections, asthma, bronchitis, irritable bowel syndrome and colitis.

Milk and Diabetes

New research suggests that insulin dependent diabetes or IDDM in children is directly related to milk consumption. A specific albumin protein isolated in milk is believed to be the culprit. After a glass of milk is consumed albumin protein is directly absorbed from the intestines into circulation. Once in the blood system it ellicits an allergic reaction. The immune system responds by producing antibodies to the albumin. However, the antibodies produced to this protein are very similar to the protein molecules in the cells of the pancreas that produce insulin. The body makes a simple mistake and can't distinguish between the albumin from milk and the protein on the surface of the pancreas cells. The immune system literally attacks the insulin producing cells on the pancreas in an effort to rid itself of these large protein molecules in milk. This mistake shuts down insulin production and diabetes develops. Researchers conclude that insulin dependent diabetes is a result of genetic predisposition and excess milk consumption.

Milk Fat

Milk is very high in fat. Forty-eight percent of the total calories of one glass of whole milk is from milk fat. Thirty-one percent of the total calories of one glass of 2% milk is from milk fat. Fifteen percent of the total calories of one glass of 1% milk is from milk fat. Five percent of the total calories of one glass of skim milk is from milk fat.

One glass of 2% milk weighs 240 grams and contains 145 calories. 2% milk means that 2% of the 240 grams is from milk fat. This translates to 5 grams of milk fat in one 240 grams glass of 2% milk. One gram of fat is equal to 9 calories. Therefore 5 grams/1 glass 2% milk x 9 calories/ 1 gram of fat = 45 calories. Forty-five out of the 145 calories in one glass of 2% milk is from milk fat. This translates to 31% fat content by weight.

Vitamins and Minerals

One cup or 250 ml of 1% milk contains 11% the recommended daily intake (RDA) of vitamin A, 44% the RDA of vitamin D, 8% of the RDA of vitamin B1, 25% of the RDA of vitamin B2, 10% of the RDA of B3, 11% of the RDA of vitamin B5, 6% of the RDA of vitamin B6, 6% of the RDA of folic acid, 45% of the RDA of vitamin B12, 29% of the RDA of calcium, 23% of the RDA of phosphorus, 14% of the RDA of magnesium and 11% of the RDA of zinc.

Herbicides, Pesticides and other Toxins

Cows that produce milk consume grass and feed that is frequently contaminated with pesticides, herbicides and insecticides. These chemicals are concentrated in cow's tissue and passed on to cow's milk. Other chemical contaminants and waste products including DDT are found in trace amounts in cow's milk. Milking cows frequently develop mastitis that is treated with antibiotics including penicillin. Trace amounts of antibiotics are frequently found in milk. Milk is also frequently contaminated with viruses. Approximately 20% of cows are infected with a leukemia-type virus that is passed on through cow's milk. The implications of consuming a glass of milk contaminated with a cancer-causing virus is quite alarming. In an effort to increase cow reproduction a majority of dairy cows that produce milk are pregnant. This leads to high levels of circulating hormones such as progesterone. Milk is frequently contaminated with elevated levels of progesterone. The long term effects of consuming progesterone on the human body is not known. Progesterone may be broken down into the hormone testosterone and other androgen hormones that are known to aggravate acne and other skin problems. Excess milk consumption will only aggravate teenage acne.

Osteoporosis

Osteoporosis is a disease of older adults that causes bones to become abnormally brittle and break much easier than normal. We are constantly advised that we should increase our daily calcium intake to prevent osteoporosis. We are told that milk is a great source of dietary calcium and we should drink milk daily to help prevent osteoporosis. However, there are problems with this simplistic approach.

Calcium and Phosphorus

The recommended daily intake of calcium is 800 to 1200 mg per day. One cup or 250 ml of 1% milk contains 300 mg of calcium. Milk is a good source of calcium, but also is a high source of phosphorus. Phosphorus is a mineral that normally occurs with calcium in many of the foods we consume. About 80% of phosphorus is contained in bones and teeth.

The calcium to phosphorus ratio is important in predicting the bioavailability of dietary calcium. In human milk the calcium to phosphorus ratio is about 2:1. In cow's milk this ratio decreases to 1.2:1. The low calcium to phosphorus ratio of cow's milk means that there are almost equal amounts of calcium and phosphorus. Excess phosphorus removes calcium from bones. Phosphorus combines with calcium to form calcium phosphates. Calcium phosphates are removed from the body and excreted in the urine. Therefore, a high phosphorus intake promotes calcium loss in urine. Eventhough milk is a good source of calcium, the proportionally high source of phosphorus limits its availability to build healthy bones.

Homogenization

It is the current belief of many respected scientists and doctors that the consumption of homogenized milk directly promotes atherosclerosis or hardening of the arteries.

Homogenization is the commercial process in which whole milk is mixed together to produce a homogenous fluid of uniform texture. Whole milk is composed of a larger portion of whey and a smaller portion of cream. Whey is the the thin, salty fluid that is usually discarded after cheese and butter are made. Cream is the thick, rich fluid that is used to make butter and cheese. Whey is a bland, watery fluid that doesn't taste good to most people. Cream is primarily composed of fat and tastes good to most people. Cream is much heavier than whey and the two constituents don't mix well together. Homogenization is the process where the two different constituents of milk are mixed together to produce a great tasting drink.

In its natural state, fat from the cream contains very large molecules that can't pass through the wall of the intestines. These fat molecules must be broken down by normal digestive processes before they are absorbed into the body. During the process of homogenization these large fat molecules are broken down into smaller fat molecules so they can mix easily with whey. These small fat molecules form little droplets of fat called micelles. These micelles don't need to be broken down by normal enzymes in the gut and they bypass the normal digestive process. Micelles are directly absorbed into the body.

Xanthine Oxidase

When we light a fire we burn logs to produce heat and energy. The ashes left over are metabolic byproducts of this process. They cannot be reburned and are considered waste products that are usually discarded. Xanthine is a normal byproduct of metabolism produced in many mammals. Xanthine is like the ashes produced from a fire. The body tries to get rid of this waste product as it accumulates. The body uses an enzyme called xanthine oxidase to break down xanthine into another waste product called uric acid that is then removed from the body. Milk normally contains a small quantity of xanthine oxidase. When we drink unhomogenized milk xanthine oxidase is digested and broken down in the intestines. However, during the process of homogenization xanthine oxidase mixes with milk fat and becomes incorporated into the micelles. These micelles which are small enough to escape digestion are directly absorbed into the body. Once absorbed into the blood the micelles release xanthine oxidase into circulation. The free enzyme can then damage the delicate inner lining of the blood vessel wall. The damage to the blood vessel wall creates a roughened surface to which circulating cholesterol in the blood can attach. Atherosclerosis or hardening of the arteries is then promoted.

Patient files

After exhausting conventional medical therapies a distraught mother brought Matthew T. a 2 year old child to our clinic. Matthew suffered from frequent colds and flus. He was always nasally congested and produced a lot of mucous and phlegm. He had dark rings around his eyes. Colds frequently developed into ear infections. He was always prescribed antibiotics that helped clear the immediate infection, but mucous, phlegm and infections would return. Matthew also suffered from stomach aches and frequent attacks of diarrhea. Upon questioning his mother she stated that she breast fed her son until 5 months. She weaned him on formula and cow's milk. After reviewing his daily diet it was revealed that he consumed a large amount of milk, cheese and other dairy products. We advised the mother to discontinue use of all dairy products. Instead she was advised to use goat's milk, nut milks, rice milk, soy milk and tofu milk as an alternative to cow's milk. We prescribed a few supplements to help stimulate Matthew's immune system. After two months of being placed on dairy restriction he had experienced no infections and had significantly decreased amounts of mucous and phlegm.

Rose A. was a 29 year old legal secretary who experienced periodic episodes of abdominal bloating, gas, flatulence and mucous diarrhea. She was previously worked up by a gastroenterologist who diagnosed her with irritable bowel syndrome. She wasn't satisfied with the diagnosis and sought help at our clinic. After reviewing her diet it was revealed that she consumed 2 glasses of skim milk, 1/2 cup of yogurt and 1 to 2 slices of low fat cheese per day. We performed a food allergy test to determine offending foods. It was confirmed that she was sensitive to all constituents of cow's milk. We advised her to discontinue all dairy products and use appropriate substitutes. After following our advise she felt significantly better and had experienced much less episodes of gas, bloating and diarrhea. She has even noticed that her skin has cleared up.

13

Salt

Salt is essential for life in small to moderate amounts. However, it can cause many health problems in large amounts. In North America we consume twenty to forty times more salt than is needed. Excess salt consumption is related to many common disorders including high blood pressure, swelling edema and heart disease. These conditions can be improved or alleviated by reducing daily salt intake.

Problems associated with excess salt consumption include abdominal bloating, breast tenderness, constipation, edema, fatigue, electrolyte imbalance, frequent urination, headaches, hemorrhoids, high blood pressure, hypertension, kidney disease, muscle weakness, premenstrual syndrome, tinnitus or ringing in the ears and swelling around the extremities including the wrists, hands, ankles and feet. The problem with salt consumption is that many people simply consume way too much of it.

Salt Structure and Function

Salt is a simple chemical that contains sodium and chloride. We need small amounts of salt to be healthy. Sodium is the major positive electrolyte and chloride is the major negative electrolyte in blood. There is only very small amounts of salt inside cells. Most salt is contained in the blood and extracellular fluid. Sodium and chloride are involved in pH regulation and help to buffer the blood from being too acidic or too alkaline. Sodium and chloride are also intimately involved in the nervous system and nerve conduction. Thirty to 45% of salt is contained in bone. Sodium and chloride combine with calcium, fluoride and potassium to create hard salts that are responsible, in part, for giving bones their hardness.

Salt Deficiency and Excess

Salt deficiency probably never occurs. Salt is contained in so many different foods that inadequate dietary intake is unlikely. However, low blood sodium and chloride levels can occur as a result of certain medical conditions. Salt requirements increase during periods of pregnancy and stress. Salt toxicity can occur as a result of excess salt intake. The regular salt intake of some North Americans approaches 50% of the toxic dose. Excess salt intake is associated with many serious medical conditions. Salt restriction should be practiced by all individuals with high blood pressure, edema, swelling and heart disease.

Recommended Daily Allowance

The recommended daily allowance of salt is 1000 to 3000 mg per day. Many well respected physicians and scientists contend that the RDA is much too high. Humans need a minimum daily salt intake of 500 mg per day. A more desirable and attainable salt intake would be 500 to 1000 mg per day. Many North American people routinely consume 10,000 to 20,000 mg of salt per day or twenty to forty times the minimum daily salt intake.

Salt and Sodium

Approximately 40% of salt is sodium and 60% chloride by weight. Therefore, 1000 mg of salt contains about 400 mg of sodium and 600 mg of chloride. One teaspoon of table salt contains 5000 mg of salt and 2000 mg of sodium. One half teaspoon of table salt contains 2500 mg of salt and 1000 mg of sodium. One quarter teaspoon of salt contains 1250 mg of salt and 500 mg of sodium. One quarter teaspoon of salt per day supplies the minimum daily salt intake. Many North Americans routinely consume in excess of four teaspoons of salt per day. Salt and sodium content are often used interchangeably. Sodium content is now used much more commonly on labels and package inserts than salt levels. We will continue to refer to sodium levels instead of salt levels.

Salt Preservatives and Additives

Salt is often listed as a common ingredient in many foods. It occurs both naturally and as an additive. Salt is a natural preservative that is added to many foods to prevent breakdown by bacteria. Salt was used to cure foods by our ancestors so they could eat a variety of foods during the harsh winter months. Salt continues to be one of the most common food additives. Large levels of salt are routinely added to many refined and processed foods.

Natural Sources of Sodium

Common natural sources of sodium include table salt, fish, seafoods, chicken, beef, pork, other animal meats, eggs, milk, cheese. Organs meats such as liver, kidney and shellfish are higher in sodium content than other meats and fish. It is interesting to note that saltwater fish contains no more sodium content than freshwater fish. Most vegetables contain a small amount of sodium. Grains and cereals contain a small amount of sodium. Most fruits contain only trace amounts of sodium. Regular tapwater can contain significant amounts of sodium. Hardness of water refers to the amount of dissolved minerals in the water. Sodium is one of the main minerals responsible for giving water its hardness. You can find out the sodium content of your drinking water by contacting appropriate government authorities in your community.

Other Sources of Sodium

Other compounds in which sodium is an additive include sodium bicarbonate used to make bread rise, baking soda used to make bread rise, brine used as a preservative, disodium phosphate used an emulsifier to thicken foods, monosodium phosphate as a seasoning and flavor enhancer, sodium acetate used to control pH, sodium alginate used to thicken ice cream, sodium ascorbate used as a form of vitamin C, sodium aluminum sulphate used as a bleaching agent, sodium calcium alginate used to thicken ice cream and chocolate milk, sodium citrate used to control pH, sodium diacetate used as a preservative, sodium erythorbate used as a preservative, sodium hydroxide used in food processing, sodium nitrate used to preserve meats, sodium propionate used to inhibit molds in foods, sodium sorbate used as a preservative, sodium stearyl fumarate used as a bleaching agent and sodium sulphite used as a preservative on dried fruits and vegetables.

Hidden Salt

Most of the salt we consume is hidden in foods we eat. Seventy-seven percent of daily salt intake is contained in processed and refined foods.

The salt is already added to canned, packaged and preserved foods that we buy in the supermarket or eat in a restaurant. Only 11% of daily salt intake is from the salt we add to food. Many people erroneously believe that salt restriction means not using the salt shaker to salt foods. This assumption is ridiculous and a poor method of salt restriction. Salt restriction should focus on limiting refined and processed foods that we consume. Remember, most of the salt we consume is hidden in the foods we eat.

Sodium Content of Common Beverages and Foods

Item	Milligrams Sodium
Water (fresh ground water)	0-80
Fruit (fresh)	0-5
Fruit (canned)	0-5
Fruit (juice)	0-5
Vegetables (fresh)	0-50
Vegetables (frozen)	0-50
Vegetables (canned)	200-500
Vegetables (fresh juice)	100-300
Vegetable Juice (Canned Tomato or V-8 juice)	200-400
Milk 1% (12 ounces)	122
Milk 2% (12 ounces)	122
Cheese - Cheddar (1 ounce)	140-200
Cheese - Feta (1 ounce)	350-450
Cheese - Mozzarella (1 ounce)	75-200
Cream of Wheat (1 ounce)	0-8
Oat Bran Cereal (1 ounce)	0-3
Instant Apple/Cinnamon Oatmeal (1 ounce)	100-200
Corn Flakes (1 ounce)	250-300
Rice Crispies (1 ounce)	250-300
Pasta noodles (1 serving)	0-5
Rice (1 ounce)	0-5
Potato (1 medium)	0-20
Potato Chips - Old Dutch BBQ (1 ounce)	350-400
Peanuts - unsalted (1 ounce)	0-10
Peanuts - salted (1 ounce)	100-300
Peanut butter - regular (2 tbsp)	150-400
Kraft Miracle Whip (1 tbsp)	200-300
Kraft Oil and Vinegar Dressing (1 tbsp)	200-300
Kraft Thousand Island Dressing (1 tbsp)	150-250
Beef - regular ground (1 ounce)	20-40

Pork - regular ground (1 ounce)	20-40
Chicken (1 ounce)	20-40
Salmon - (3 ounces)	40-80
Trout (3 ounces)	30-60
Bologna (1 ounce)	150-300
Pastrami (1 ounce)	200-300
Salami (1 ounce)	200-400
Arby's Roast Beef Sandwich (Super)	798
McDonald's Big Mac Sandwich	890
McDonald's Cheeseburger Sandwich	725
McDonald's Filet-O-Fish Sandwich	730
McDonald's McChicken Sandwich	830
McDonald's French Fries (large)	200
Wendy's Big Classic Sandwich	1058

High Blood Pressure

Hypertension or high blood pressure is defined as blood pressure in your arteries and veins greater than 140/90 millimeters of mercury on three or more different readings. By comparison your car tire in your automobile has approximately 30 to 40 millimeters of mercury of pressure.

Your heart and blood vessel system comprise a closed system. The human body has an incredible network of arteries, capillaries and veins. If you lined up every artery, capillary and vein there is an estimated one thousand miles of blood vessels. Your heart pumps blood through your arteries to distant parts of the body. In very small vessels called capillaries fluid and nutrients are exchanged to all cells of your body. The remaining fluid returns to the heart in veins back to the heart and the whole cycle is repeated. Blood pressure readings are given as two numbers. The two numbers reflect different pressure in the blood vessels at different times. When your heart contracts it forces blood out into the blood vessels at high pressure. This is the top number or the systolic pressure. The average systolic pressure should be 120 millimeters of mercury or approximately three times the pressure in your car tire. When the heart relaxes there is still pressure in your blood vessels. Remember your heart and blood vessels comprise a closed system. The bottom number is the diastolic pressure. The average diastolic pressure should be 80 millimeters of mercury or two times the pressure in your car tire.

High blood pressure is estimated to affect 20 to 40% of the North American population or up to 60 million people. It occurs equally males and females and occurs twice as common in black people as it does in white people. The cause of high blood pressure is not entirely known. Current evidence suggests that an imbalance between electrolytes in blood is the main cause. High levels of sodium and low levels of calcium, magnesium and potassium can cause elevated blood pressure. Blood pressure is usually tightly regulated in the body between fluid in the blood, primarily water, and electrolytes, primarily sodium in the blood. When we consume a high level of sodium the blood absorbs the sodium and reflects a corresponding high level. The unnaturally increased sodium level in the blood fools the body into believing it is low in water. The body tries to conserve water and increase fluid volume in the blood. The kidneys stop releasing so much water in urine, the intestines are robbed of any water that remains after digestion and the sweat cells in the skin shut down. The net result is that water is retained in the blood to balance the high sodium levels. High blood pressure develops and is a direct consequence of high sodium intake in our diet.

Most people are not even aware that they have high blood pressure. Hypertension is often considered a silent disease and does not produce any symptoms at all. Symptoms such as dizzinesss, flushed face, headaches, nose bleed, anxiety, stress and nervousness are not due to elevated blood pressure. Direct consequences of having high blood pressure include swelling, edema, fluid overload, congestive heart failure, brain hemorrhage, aneurysm or rupture of a blood vessel and a stroke. Uncontrolled high blood pressure often ends with fatal results.

High Blood Pressure and Salt Restriction

Lowering salt intake lowers blood pressure in almost all individuals with hypertension. At least 60% of people with elevated blood pressure can significantly lower the readings by reducing salt intake. Approximately 25% of all individuals with high blood pressure are sodium sensitive. This means that their high salt intake is the direct cause of the high blood pressure. For the remaining 75% of individuals with high blood pressure there are other factors beside salt intake responsible for their elevated readings. However, all people with hypertension can benefit from sodium restriction. One study of over 10,000 people in 32 different countries showed that no individuals with a sodium intake less than 1500 mg per day had high blood pressure. As people consumed more salt their blood pressure readings got consistently higher.

It is important to note that elevated blood sodium is not the only cause of high blood pressure. Corresponding low levels of other minerals including calcium, magnesium and potassium consistently go along with high levels of sodium. Decreasing sodium intake and increasing calcium, magnesium and potassium would be a wise approach in controlling blood pressure.

Edema, Fluid Retention and Swelling

Edema, fluid retention and swelling in the body can be directly related to the sodium intake of our diet. An elevated sodium intake not only increases the sodium content of the blood but also increases the sodium content of the fluid between cells. The fluid between the billions of cells of our body is called extracellular fluid. It is primarily composed of water, minerals, electrolytes and nutrients. Sodium content of the extracellular fluid affects the water content. A high sodium level fools the body into believing that the water content of extracellular fluid is low. Consequently, water is conserved in the extracellular fluid and edema, fluid retention and swelling develop.

Sodium Restriction

Sodium restriction means more than not using the salt shaker to salt foods you eat. Sodium restriction means that we should read labels for sodium content and actively decrease our sodium intake in foods we eat. Remember that a significant proportion of sodium we consume is hidden in the refined and processed foods. This means we should restrict our intake of refined and processed foods. Any food that contains more than 400 mg of sodium per serving is considered a high sodium food and its use in our diet should be restricted.

Patient Files

Theresa F. was a 38 year old bank clerk who suffered from fatigue, fluid retention, abdominal bloating, swelling around her wrists and ankles, headaches and constipation. A routine blood test was unremarkable. Blood pressure was high normal. She consumed only 1 to 2 cups of coffee per day. She ate a relatively healthy diet with moderate amounts of chicken and fish, whole grains, fresh fruits and vegetables. She consumed a daily regimen of vitamins and minerals. After further questioning she stated that she often craved salt and would use salt at most meals. We calculated her sodium intake as 10,000 mg per day. We placed her on a low sodium diet. We advised her to discontinue salting her foods, read labels for sodium content and generally avoid all foods high in salt. Within 3 weeks of sodium restriction her fluid retention and swelling significantly decreased. Her headaches diminished and she was experiencing regular bowel movements.

Mike D. was a 52 year old insurance executive who presented at our clinic with high blood pressure. He was slightly overweight, had marginally high cholesterol and smoked 1/2 pack of cigarettes per day. His blood pressure reading was about 160/95 on three separate occasions. He often consumed fried and processed foods, frequently ate at fast food restaurants and ate peanuts, beef jerky, potato chips and other highly salted foods. After reviewing his dietary habits we determined his salt intake to be 16,000 mg per day. We strongly advised him to make some simple dietary changes. Avoid all refined and processed foods and increase consumption of whole grains, fresh fruits and vegetables. Additionally, he would have to avoid salt and salted foods. We recommended several supplements including a calcium, magnesium and potassium supplement. In two weeks we rechecked his blood pressure and it was 140/85. After two months his blood pressure was 130/85 and he felt younger and much more energetic.

14

Sugar

Sugar is a simple sweet tasting chemical that is used to produce energy in the body. Sugar is naturally found in many different foods including grains, cereals, starchy vegetables and fruit. Sugar is also added to many refined and processed foods.

Problems associated with sugar consumption include abdominal pains, allergies, anxiety, bed-wetting, bloating, breast tenderness, candidiasis, colds, cravings for sweets, crying bouts, dental cavities, depression, diabetes mellitus, diarrhea, dizziness, epilepsy, flu, excessive sweating, fainting, fatigue, flatulence, gingivitis or gum disese, headaches, heart disease, heart palpitations, high cholesterol level, high triglyceride level, hives, hyperactivity, hypoglycemia or low blood sugar, infection, insomnia, irritability, irritable bowel syndrome, itching, kidney stones, lightheadness, menstrual cramps and pain, moodiness and mood swings, muscle aches and weakness, nausea, obesity, overweight, osteoporosis, poor concentration, poor memory, premenstrual syndrome, rapid heart beat, seizures, skin rashes, vaginal itching, vaginitis, weakness and yeast infection.

Carbohydrates

Sugar belongs to a family of related chemicals called carbohydrates. A carbohydrate is a class of foods that contains carbon, hydrogen and oxygen in certain specific ratios. Carbohydrates occur naturally in both plants and animals. Carbohydrates are an important source of immediate energy for the human body. One gram of carbohydrates furnishes the body with 4 calories of energy. Carbohydrates are present, at least in small amounts, in most foods.

Sugars and Starches

The two main forms of carbohydrates are sugars and starches. Sugars are small, simple molecules while starches are large, complex sugars. Sugars usually contain one or two simple molecules while starches usually contain at least ten or more molecules attached together. Monosaccharides contain only one sugar molecule. Monosaccharides include glucose or dextrose derived from grape sugar, fructose or fruit sugar and galactose which is derived from milk sugar. Disaccharides are double sugars that contain two sugar molecules attached together. Disaccharides include sucrose which is found in sugar canes or sugar beets, maltose or malt sugar, lactose or milk sugar.

All ripe fruits and many vegetables contain natural sugars. Grains and cereals such as wheat, rye, oats, rice and starchy vegetables such as potatoes, beans and squash contain starches. Sugars are usually burned for fuel by the body shortly after they are consumed. They may also be stored in the body in the form of glycogen for later use. If sugars are consumed in excessive amounts the body changes them into fats and triglycerides which are stored throughout the body.

Refined White Sugar

Refined white sugar is considered an empty food that only furnishes the body with energy. Sugars in nature usually occur along with other nutrients. White sugar contains no vitamins, no minerals and no fiber. Natural sugars such as honey, molasses and pure maple syrup contain many different vitamins and minerals. One teaspoon of honey contains small amounts of calcium, magnesium and vitamin C. One teaspoon of molasses contains 44 milligram of calcium, 1 milligram of iron and 175 milligram of potassium. Honey, molasses and other natural sweeteners also contain trace amounts of many other vitamins and minerals. White sugar, on-the-other-hand, contains no vitamins and no minerals.

Commercially Available Sugar

All commercially available white sugar is derived from either sugar beets or sugar cane. White table sugar is primarily sucrose. Brown sugar is simply white sugar that has been coated with molasses to give it a darkened appearance. Milk sugar is derived from the processing of milk. Milk sugar is primarily all lactose. Honey is derived from the honey bee which collects sugars from varous plants. Molasses and malt sugar are derived from grains and cereals. Maple syrup is derived from the sap of various trees. Fruit sugar is the sugar that is derived from processing different fruits. Date sugar is derived from raw dates All commercially available fruit sugar is corn sugar. Corn sugar is derived from the partial breakdown of corn starch from corn.

Sugar Consumption

The problem with sugar is that we simply eat too much of it. A small amount of sugar is vital for life and necessary for energy production. However, excess consumption of sugar has harmful effects throughout the human body. Sugar consumption has rapidly increased in the twentieth century. Our ancestors consumed very little refined sugar compared to the quantities we now consume. Prior to 1800 the average sugar consumption was estimated to be less that 9 kilograms or 20 pounds per year. In 1900 the average sugar consumption was estimated to be between 14 and 18 kilograms or 30 and 40 pounds per year. By 1990 the average sugar consumption is estimated to be between 55 and 64 kilograms or 120 and 140 pounds per year. The average North American consumes 150 grams of sugar per day. As mentioned earlier, one gram of carbohydrates produces 4 calories of energy. The average daily consumption of sugar produces 600 calories of energy. If we consider that the average daily caloric intake is 2000 calories then 30% of our daily caloric intake is from sugar.

Hidden Sugar

Sugar is often added to many refined and processed foods. Seventy-five percent of all sugar we eat is allready added to foods we buy at the supermarket or eat at a restaurant. Like salt, sugar is hidden in many foods. Only 25% of sugar is added to foods directly. Large amounts of sugar are added to many common household foods. Breakfast cereals, jams and jellies, ketchup, salad dressings, chocolate milk, ice cream, yogurt, canned vegetables and fruit, soft drinks, fruit drinks, candy, chocolate, cookies, cakes, pies, doughnuts, jello are common sources of large amounts of hidden sugar. Just read the label. Sugar is also added to many vitamins and medicines commonly prescribed by doctors and available at the local pharmacy. Many common over-the-counter or OTC medicines including Actifed syrup, Chlor-Trimeton, Dimetapp elixir, Benylin syrup and Robitussin syrup contain anywhere from 15 to 80% sugar. Sugar is often added to these medicines to make them taste good, especially for children.

Sugar Content of Common Beverages and Foods

Item	Teaspoons Sugar
All Bran Cereal (1ounce)	1.3
Cap'n Crunch (1 ounce)	3.0
Cheerios (1 ounce)	0.3
Corn Flakes (1 ounce)	0.5
Honey Smacks (1 ounce)	4.0
Life Cereal (1 ounce)	1.3
Puffed Wheat (1 ounce)	0
Rice Krispies (1 ounce)	0.8
Shredded Wheat (1 ounce)	0.3
Milk 2% (1 ounce)	0.4
Chocolate Milk (1 cup)	2.7
Chocolate bar (2 ounces)	8.0
Hard Candy (2 ounces)	8.0
Doughnut (1 commercial)	6.0
Cupcake (1 commercial)	6.0
Hamburger bun (1 commercial)	3.0
Yogurt - flavored (1 cup)	4.1
Ice Cream - vanilla flavored (1 cup)	6.4
Sherbet (1/2 cup)	6.0
Popsicle - flavored (1)	4.5
Chocolate Pudding (1/2 cup)	5.3
Pears - canned with syrup (1/2 cup)	3.6
Pineapple - canned (1/2 cup)	3.0
Soft Drink (12 ounces)	8.0
Kool-Aid (8 ounces)	6.0
Tang (8 ounes)	4.0
Orange Hi-C (8 ounces)	5.0

Sugar Addiction

Do you have a sweet tooth? Do you crave sugar, chocolate or other sweets? Do you have to eat sweets or chocolate everyday? Do you eat one or more candy bars per week or per day? Do you eat sweets to comfort yourself? Do you eat sweets at work or at home? Do sugar cravings interfere with your normal relationships at home or at work? Do sugar cravings disrupt your life? If you've answered yes to one or more of the following questions then you may be addicted to sugar. The problem with sugar is that it tastes so good. Sugar stimulates taste buds in our mouth and tongue. Once the taste buds are stimulated they send electrical impulses to the brain. And our brain tells us that sugar tastes sweet.

Current research indicates that sugar addiction may be more than a psychological addiction. Glucose, a simple sugar, is the main food that is utalized by the brain and nervous system. Excess sugar consumption increases glucose levels in the brain. High levels of glucose alters chemicals in the brain called neurotransmitters. Imbalances of specific neurotransmitters can cause physiological addiction. High levels of glucose stimulates the production of highly addictive opiods and enkephalins. High levels of glucose decrease the amounts of other neurotransmitters including dopamine, GABA and serotonin. These chemicals affect an area of the brain called the limbic system. The limbic system is an area of the brain that is responsible for certain aspects of emotion and behavior. Elevated levels of opiods and enkephalins stimulates pleasure areas in the limbic system of the brain. Withdrawal of glucose decreases opiods and enkephalins and causes physiological addiction.

Diabetes

Diabetes mellitus is a condition characterized by abnormally high levels of blood sugar. Five to 10% of the North American population suffer from diabetes. The most common of diabetes is non-insulin dependent diabetes (NIDDM) or adult onset diabetes. Approximately 90% of diabetics suffer from non-insulin dependent diabetes. Insulin dependent diabetes (IDDM) or juvenile onset diabetes has its onset in childhood or early adulthood. Approximately 10% of diabetics suffer from insulin dependent diabetes. Diabetes is usually due to an abnormality with insulin. Insulin is a small hormone produced in the pancreas. Insulin is released into the blood in response to a rise in blood sugar levels. Insulin stimulates the cells of the body to absorb sugar from the blood and thereby reduce high sugar levels in the blood. Insulin dependent diabetes is strictly due to a genetic abnormality in the production of insulin. Non-insulin dependent diabetes is associated with an abnormality of insulin production, abnormal release of insulin from the pancreas or a sensitivity of the body to the hormone.

There is a strong association between obesity and the development of non-insulin diabetes. The majority of NIDDM individuals are overweight, lead a sedentary lifestyle and have a high caloric intake that is especially high in sugar and other refined carbohydrates. Excess sugar consumption is directly associated with the development of non-insulin dependent diabetes. High levels of sugar in the blood constantly stress the pancreas to produce insulin. Like any organ or gland the pancreas can become overworked and over-stressed. The regulation of the pancreas becomes affected. The gland may produce inappropriate amounts of insulin in response to different blood sugar levels. An under-production of insulin in response to sugar in the blood leads to elevated blood sugar levels. An overproduction of insulin may result in the body becoming sensitized to the abnormally high hormone levels. High levels of insulin are produced in response to high levels of blood sugar. The cells of the body become sensitized to the high levels of insulin and constantly need large amounts of the hormone for normal uptake of sugar from the blood. The normal regulation of blood sugar by insulin from the pancreas becomes chaotic. Excess consumption of sugar is directly responsible for abnormal blood sugar levels.

Hypoglycemia

Hypoglycemia or low blood sugar is the presence of abnormally low levels of blood sugar. Symptoms of hypoglycemia include nervousness, irritability, faintness, weakness, muscle weakness, tremors and shakes, heart palpitations, rapid heart rate, increased blood pressure, tingling in the skin, hunger, sweating, dizziness, lack of balance, blurred vision headaches, cold hands and feet, anxiety, depression, mood swings and an inability to concentrate. Ten to 25% of the North American population is believed to suffer from varying degrees of hypoglycemia. Hypoglycemia is the result of an excessive rate of removal of sugar from the blood or a decreased release of sugar into the blood. Overproduction of insulin or an overdose and abnormally low blood sugar levels can cause hypoglycemia.

Immune Depression

Excess sugar consumption depresses immune system function. The effect of sugar on the immune system is believed to be due to the structural similarity of many sugars and vitamin C. Simple sugars or monosaccharides are composed of a six carbon backbone. Vitamin C also shares the six carbon backbone. Both sugar and vitamin C share the same transport site that allows them to get in white blood cells. Sugar competes with vitamin C at these transport sites. High levels of sugar saturates all the binding sites and prevents vitamin C from entering white blood cells. Sugar impairs the ability of white blood cells to engulf and destroy foreign bacteria and viruses. High doses of sugar literally paralyzes a specific white blood called a neutrophil. Under normal circumstances neutrophils engulf and digest microbes in the human body. High levels of sugar in the blood prevents neutrophils from doing their job. High levels of sugar depress the function of another white blood cell called a lymphocyte. Certain lymphocytes regulate the function of the immune system while other lymphocytes produce antibodies. Sugar consumption should be sharply discontinued at the onset of any infection.

Candida and Chronic Yeast Infection

Candidiasis and chronic yeast infection has reached epidemic proportions in recent years. Our excess sugar consumption is responsible for a large part of this problem. Yeast are small organisms that have relatively simple digestive systems. Yeast can't digest and breakdown complex foods and must rely on sugar as the primary source of energy. Yeast directly feed off the sugar we put in our stomach. Eating more sugar only feeds the microbes and can lead to a whole host of problems that are legion with this infection.

Artificial Sweeteners

Artificial sweetener are synthetic chemicals that look and taste like sugar. They are usually very low in calories and are often preferred by dieters instead of sugar.

Aspartame

Aspartame or Nutrasweet is a synthetic natural sweetener that is made artificially. Aspartame is made from methyl alcohol and two amino acids, aspartic acid and phenylalanine. The presence of phenylalanine in this substance poses a serious problem for a few individuals who cannot breakdown the amino acid. The inability to break down phenylalanine results in high levels throughout the body. A condition known as phenylketonuria results. If left unchecked it may cause mental retardation and other abnormalities. The U.S. and Canadian governments require that aspartame is properly labelled to warn those individuals with this rare disorder that this product contains phenylalanine. Aspartame is generally regarded as safe for consumption by the majority of the population. However, aspartame has been associated with the development of health problems in some individuals. Problems associated with excess aspartame consumption include allergies, asthma, depression, dizziness, fainting, headaches, hives, memory impairment, menstrual pains, mood swings, nausea, seizures and skin rashes.

Chocolate

Chocolate is widely consumed throughout the world. In North America we consume more chocolate than most other countries combined. Chocolate is produced from seeds obtained from the cocoa plant that grows in tropical climates throughout the world. Unrefined cocoa powder contains 5% sugar and 23% fat. Cocoa powder also contains small amounts of caffeine and theobromine which have stimulant effects on the body. Sugar is added to cocoa powder to produce refined chocolate. As much 50% of the calories from chocolates and candy bars comes from sugar. Most of the remaining calories comes from fat. Chocolate has very few vitamins, minerals and nutrients.

Carob

Carob is often used as a chocolate substitute available in most health food stores. Carob is produced from the pods of the carob plant that grows in tropical climates. Carob contains no cocoa. Carob powder used commercially is very high in sugar. Carob powder is much higher in sugar than cocoa powder. Refined carob powder contains up to 48% sugar. Additional sugar is often addded to carob bars and candies. Be wary of so called "natural" substitutes available in health food stores. They are nothing more than chocolate free sugar substitutes.

Fructose

Fructose is a simple sugar that naturally occurs in most fruits, honey and corn sugar. Fructose is often added to refined and processed foods. It is used as a substitute to glucose and sucrose. It is often added to fruit drinks and soft drinks. Most commercially available fructose comes from corn in the form of corn syrup. Many people who are sensitive or allergic to corn or corn should be wary of commercially available fructose. Problems associated with excess fructose consumption includes abdominal bloating, allergies, asthma, diarrhea, eczema, gas, indigestion and skin rashes.

Saccharin

Saccharin is an artificial chemical that was first produced in 1879 and was used for more than sixty years. Saccharin is a white, crystalline coal-tar compound used as a sugar substitute. The popularity of saccharin was limited due to its unpleasant, bitter aftertaste. The long term safety of this substance remains controversial. Certain studies associate excess saccharin consumption with the development of certain cancers including bladder cancer. Its safety for pregnant women is also questionable and remains controversial. Saccharin was banned in Canada in 1977, but remains available in the United States.

Sorbitol

Sorbitol is a sugar that is found naturally in various berries and fruits. Most commercially available sorbitol is produced artificially. Sorbitol is converted by the body to glucose or fructose. Sorbitol has the same caloric value as other sugars. High levels of sorbitol are found in the lens of the eye of diabetics and is related to the development of cataracts. A 50% sorbitol solution is used as a diuretic. Problems associated with excess sorbitol consumption include abdominal bloating, abdominal cramps, diarrhea, gas, indigestion and irritable bowel syndrome.

Patient Files

Johnny S. was a pleasant six year old child that was brought to our clinic with his concerned parents. His parents explained that Johnny had trouble concentrating in school, disrupted the class frequently and had a poor attention span. Their family doctor believed that Johnny showed classic signs of hyperactivity or attention deficit disorder. He suggested that they administer the child a drug called Ritalin to help control his behavior. However, they decided to get another opinion. After reviewing the the child's dietary habits it was revealed that he consumed far too much sugar and refined carbohydrates. A food sensitivity test was administered to help identify irritating foods and chemical food additives. The child was placed on a hypo-allergenic diet and told to strictly avoid all sugar, refined carbohydrates and all foods with food additives and preservatives for one month. After one month his parents returned and were amazed at the improvement in his behavior. They reported that his attention span had improved and he experienced significantly less outbursts.

Diane R. was a 34 year old artist who presented at our clinic complaining of fatigue, moodiness, irritability, inability to concentrate, dizziness, cold hands and feet and burning skin. Symptoms were frequently worse during her premenstrual period. A routine blood test for anemia, blood sugar and low thyroid function was negative. A dietary review revealed that she consumed 2 to 3 cups of coffee, frequently missed breakfast and consumed refined and processed foods. She also indicated that chocolate was her favorite food. It was evident that Diane consumed too much sugar and refined carbohydrates. She was diagnosed with hypoglycemia. We suggested some simple lifestyle and dietary changes. We recommended that she eat three meals per day with frequent small snacks between meals. We advised her strongly avoid sugar and refined carbohydrates, eat whole grains and cereals, fresh fruits and vegetables. Additionally we recommended a few supplements including chromium. After several weeks she reported she felt significantly better. She was not fatigued, had more energy and could think much clearer.

15

Natural Foods

APPLE

The American philosopher, politician and scientist Ben Franklin was the first to popularize the old adage "an apple a day keeps the doctor away." Apples are sweet tasting fruit, rich in carbohydrates, fiber, vitamins and minerals. A medium-sized apple weighs about 200 milligrams and contains only 80 calories of energy. An average-sized apple contains 3.5 grams of fiber. About 25% of the fiber content of the apple is in the form of pectin. Pectin is a water soluble fiber that absorbs water in the intestines. Apple pectin helps to reduce cholesterol levels. The pectin in apples binds cholesterol in the small intestine before it is absorbed. Apples help to raise HDL or "good" cholesterol levels and decrease LDL or "bad" cholesterol. Apples also help to reduce blood pressure and blood sugar levels. Apples have been used as a popular treatment for both constipation and diarrhea. The high fiber content of apples is very beneficial in helping to add bulk to stool content and improve constipation. A mixture of applesauce and yogurt is a popular treatment for diarrhea. Apple fiber helps to decrease appetite and satiate hunger feelings in the stomach. Apples are a great when trying to lose weight or on a diet. Apple juice inhibits the growth of various viruses and bacteria. Pure and unsweetened apple juice may help to fight common respiratory and digestive infections. The skin of apples also contain large amounts of caffeic acid, chlorogenic acid and malic acid. These chemicals have demonstrated anti-cancer effects. A minority of individuals are sensitive to apples and cannot consume apples without having bloating, indigestion and stomach ache. Peeling the apples before they are consumed helps to make it easier to digest this fruit. Two to three medium-sized apples per day are recommended for the potent health benefits.

APRICOT

Like all yellow and orange vegetables and fruits, apricots are rich in beta-carotene. Beta-carotene is a potent anti-oxidant that helps to prevent free radical damage to the body. Beta-carotene helps to prevent free radical damage that can lead to the development of cancer. Apricots are high in potassium. Three medium-sized apricots contain 400 milligrams of potassium. The high level of potassium may be useful in reducing high blood pressure. Apricots have gained notoriety in the last several years due to the high content of amygdalin or laetrile. Laetrile was widely touted as an anti-cancer compound. The kernel of the apricot contains a small bitter tasting seed that contains laetrile. Laetrile is a cyanide containing compound that works like a natural chemotherapy agent. Cyanide is toxic to cells of the body including rapidly dividing cancer cells. However, it is easy to consume too much cyanide from apricot pits. Cyanide poisoning can cause vomiting, respiratory problems and even death. Excessive consumption of apricot kernels can supply the body with enough cyanide containing compounds to cause cyanide poisoning. The effectiveness of laetrile remains controversial.

ARTICHOKE

Artichoke is a large thistle-like perennial herb that grows up to 1 meter in height and is native to Europe, North Africa and the Canary islands. The immature flowerheads with the fleshy leaves are eaten as vegetable. Artichokes have been used in folk medicine to treat biliary tract obstruction, gallstones, liver problems, indigestion, blood sugar irregularities and hardening of the arteries. Artichokes contain cynarin and related chemicals that account for about 2.0% of the dry weight of the plant. Cynarin stimulates bile production from the liver and the regeneration of damaged liver cells. Cynarin lowers elevated cholesterol and triglyceride levels. Cynarin also has mild diuretic properties that increase fluid output in the kidneys. Artichokes are useful in treating a wide range of gall bladder and liver problems, help to reduce elevated cholesterol and triglyceride levels and reverse hardening of the arteries.

ASPARAGUS

Asparagus was once widely used by the Greeks and Romans as an aphrodisiac. Asparagus is rich in the B vitamins, which partly explains the effect of turning urine an orange or yellow color. Asparagus is also rich in sulfur containing compounds, such as methyl mercaptan, that further colors the urine and imparts a distinctive unpleasant odor. Asparagus is a natural diuretic that helps flush out the kidneys. Asparagus helps to reduce cholesterol levels and decrease blood pressure. Asparagus also contains appreciable amounts of the antioxidants beta-carotene, vitamin C and selenium which makes this vegetable beneficial in helping to prevent the development of cancer.

BANANA

Bananas and their cousin plantain have been widely consumed as a food in Africa, South America, India and parts of Asia. Plantain bananas have been used in Indian folk medicine for thousands of years. Plantain bananas have been used to treat abdominal bloating, indigestion, stomach inflammation, stomach ulcers and flatulence. Plantain bananas increase the production and the quality of mucous in the stomach. Mucous is a slimy, slippery substance containing sugars and protein. Mucous lines the wall of the stomach and prevents hydrochloric acid and proteolytic enzymes such as pepsin from digesting through the stomach wall. Plantain bananas have been scientifically proven to decrease stomach ulcer formation and enhance ulcer healing time. Bananas are also rich in potassium. One medium-sized banana contains about 400 milligrams of potassium. Bananas also contain no sodium and due to their high potassium content are extremely beneficial in reducing high blood pressure. Bananas are also high in fiber. One medium-sized banana contains about 3.5 grams of fiber. The water soluble pectin fiber accounts for 30% of the fiber content of the banana. The high fiber content of banana makes this fruit very beneficial in treating high blood cholesterol, constipation, diarrhea, blood sugar irregularities and obesity. The high fiber content of this fruit helps to reduce stomach pains and decrease hunger feelings.

BEANS

Beans are a broad group of vegetables including black beans, chick peas, garbanzo beans, kidney beans, lentils, lima beans, navy beans, pinto beans, split peas and white beans. Beans are rich in protein. One cup of beans contains on average of 18.0 grams of protein. Beans are good source of dietary protein for vegetarians and individuals who don't eat a lot of meat. Beans are one of the richest source of dietary fiber. One cup of beans contains an average of 6 to 7 grams of fiber. The high fiber content of beans accounts for many health benefits of this vegetable. Beans reduce total cholesterol and LDL or "bad" cholesterol levels. The fiber in beans binds cholesterol before it can be absorbed into the bloodstream. Soluble fiber lowers LDL cholesterol levels by decreasing production of cholesterol in the liver. Beans are a very good food for individuals with sugar irregularities and diabetes. The high fiber content of beans adds bulk to food in the stomach and slows the release of sugar into the intestines. The slow release of food into the intestines slows sugar absorption and prevents high blood sugar levels. This decreases insulin release in the pancreas and allows the body more time to deal with the sugar. A diet high in beans can reduce the amount of insulin needed for insulin depenedent diabetics and reduce the need for oral hypoglycemic drugs in non-insulin dependent diabetics. Beans also help to lower high blood pressure, decrease appetite and promote weight loss. The high fiber content of this food makes this vegetable useful in treating constipation. The fiber is able to bind toxins in the digestive system before they are able to be absorbed into the bloodstream. Beans also contain chemicals that inhibit the development of cancer, especially stomach, intestinal and colon cancer. Beans are also rich in complex carbohydrates and starches. One cup of beans contains an average of 50 grams of complex carbohydrates. The complex carbohydrates are composed of long chains of sugars that are only partially digested by enzymes in the digestive system. Bacteria in the gut utalize these partially digested carbohydrates for energy. As they further digest and breakdown the complex carbohydrates they produce are large amount gas. This gas is retained in the intestines causing abdominal bloating and can be later expelled as flatus. To prevent beans from producing intestinal bloating and gas soak them overnight so that water covers over the top of the beans. Discard the water and cook the soaked beans.

BLUEBERRY

Blueberries have been widely used to make jams, jellies and pies in Europe and North America for centuries. They have also been used in folk medicine to treat colds, diarrhea, hemorrhoids and varicose veins. Medicinal use bilberries, a cousin of the blueberry found in Europe, became popular in World War II when British RAF pilots consumed handfuls of these berries prior to their night flights. The pilots believed that the berries significantly improved their night vision when they flew on their missions. Blueberries are rich in a group of chemicals called anthocyanosides. Anthocyanosides range between 0.1 and 0.25% of the dry weight of the berry. Anthocyanosides have many beneficial medicinal effects including the stabilization of connective tissue around blood vessels. Anthocyanosides help to strengthen blood vessel walls. Consumption of anthocyanoside rich foods may be beneficial in treating a variety of blood vessel disorders including easy bruising, diabetic retinopathy, hemorrhoids, macular degeneration and varicose veins. Anthocyanosides have also demonstrated potent antibiotic activity against bacteria and viruses, including the polio and HIV viruses. Antibiotic activity has been demonstrated against E.coli bacteria, the most common cause of infectious diarrhea and urinary tract infections. Blueberries are also rich in tannic acid. Tannic acid is a strong astringent that binds the surface membrane of the digestive system and causes contraction of tissues. The astringent actions of tannic acid makes blueberries effective in alleviating diarrhea and reducing inflammed hemorrhoids. Blueberries contain significant amounts of fiber. One half cup or 125 milliliters of blueberries contains 2.4 grams of fiber. The high fiber content of blueberries is useful in treating high blood cholesterol, high blood pressure and blood sugar irregularities.

BROCCOLI

Broccoli is high in fiber and low in calories. One cup of cooked broccoli contains 2.4 grams of fiber and contains only 45 calories. Broccoli contains no cholesterol or fat and an insignificant amount of sodium. The high fiber content of this vegetable makes it useful in treating high blood cholesterol, constipation, blood sugar irregularities and obesity. The green color of broccoli is due to this plants high content of chlorophyll. Chlorophyll is a natural digestive system deodorant and detoxifier. Broccoli is rich in anti-cancer chemicals including carotenoids and beta-carotene, chlorophyll, dithiolthiones, glucosinolates, indoles and vitamin C. These chemicals are potent antioxidants that prevent free radical damage to the body. They effectively neutralize cancer causing chemicals and helps the body eliminate the toxic compounds. Broccoli has been scientifically proven to be effective in reducing the incidence of mouth, esophagus, stomach, intestinal, colon and rectal cancer. Broccoli also contains folic acid, iron and potassium. Broccoli and other vegetables contain chemicals called goitrogens. Goitrogens interfere with the production of thyroid hormones in the thyroid gland. A large and continual consumption of raw broccoli is not recommended for individuals with low thyroid function. Cooking broccoli inactivates the goitrogens.

CABBAGE

Fresh cabbage juice has been used for centuries to treat stomach ulcers. The effectiveness of cabbage juice in the treatment of ulcers has been attributed to its high glutamine content. Patients who consumed one liter of fresh cabbage juice per day showed remarkable improvement in the healing time of ulcers. Glutamine is believed to be involved in the production of mucous. Mucous lines the stomach wall and protects the delicate lining from the harsh effects of hydrochloric acid and proteolytic enzymes such as pepsin. Cabbage is rich anti-cancer chemicals including chlorophyll, dithiolthiones, flavonoids, indoles and isothiocyanates. These chemicals are potent antioxidants that prevent free radical damage. They effectively neutralize cancer causing chemicals and helps the body eliminate toxins. Cabbage has been scientifically proven to reduce the incidence of certain types of cancer including stomach, intestinal, colon and rectal cancer. In the laboratory, cabbage extracts have demonstrated antibiotic and antiviral effects. Other experiments have shown that cabbage extracts stimulate the production of antibodies in the immune system. Fermented cabbage or sauerkraut has multiple health benefits. Like cabbage, sauerkraut helps improve the healing time of peptic ulcers. Sauerkraut contains lactic acid which is used as a fuel source by intestinal bacteria.

CARROTS

Carrots are most commonly recommended for the development of strong eyes and good vision. Carrots were used in folk medicine to treat anxiety, asthma, bronchitis and other respiratory problems, eczema, psoriasis and other skin disorders and poor vision, decreased visual acuity, poor dark adaptation and other visual problems. Like all yellow and orange vegetables and fruits, carrots are high in carotenoids including beta-carotene. Beta-carotene is a precursor to vitamin A. One medium-sized carrot contains 80% the recommended RDA of vitamin A which is equivalent to 12,000 International Units of vitamin A. Vitamin A and beta-carotene are potent antioxidants that prevent free radical damage to the body. Antioxidants help to neutralize cancer cancer chemicals in the body. Vitamin A and beta-carotene have been scientifically proven to reduce the incidence of many types of cancer including lung cancer, stomach cancer, pancreatic cancer, intestinal cancer, colon cancer and rectal cancer. Other health benefits of vitamin A and beta-carotene include the normal growth, development and maintenance of epithelial tissue of the skin, the normal development of vision and night vision, the normal development of bones and tooth formation and can also stimulate the immune system. If you eat a lot of carrots the high beta-carotene content may turn your skin orange. This effect is transient and disappears shortly after the source of the beta-carotene is discontinued. Carrots are also high in fiber. One carrot contains 2.3 grams of fiber. The high fiber content of carrots makes this vegetable useful in treating atherosclerosis, constipation, high blood cholesterol and obesity. Carrots contain no cholesterol or fat and an insignificant amount of sodium. Carrots contains a significant amount of potassium and can help to reduce high blood pressure.

CAYENNE PEPPER

Cayenne is the strong, pungent spice obtained from the small annual shrub cultivated in tropical climates throughout the world. Cayenne has been used in folk medicine to treat asthma, bronchitis, colds, earaches, indigestion, intestinal infections, menstrual irregularities, respiratory problems, parasites, shingles and worms. It was also reported to be an aphrodisiac. Cayenne pepper contains about 2.0% of a strong oil containing the chemical capsaicin. The oil is responsible for many of the medicinal effects of this plant. Cayenne is a strong expectorant that helps to break up mucous and phlegm in the ears, nose, sinuses and lungs. Cayenne also acts as a natural decongestant. It helps to relax bronchi in the lungs and may help to treat asthma and bronchitis. Cayenne helps to lower elevated blood cholesterol and high blood pressure. Cayenne helps to thin the blood and prevent blood clots. It may be useful in treating atheroscleosis, intermittent claudication, thrombosis and strokes. Cayenne also helps to improve circulation to the hands and feet. Cayenne is a strong painkiller and has been scientifically proven to decrease nerve pain. Capsaicin helps to reduce pain by inhibitting a pain producing chemical called substance P in nerve endings throughout the body. Capsaicin is effective in reducing pain associated with diabetic neuralgia, post-surgical neuralgias, toothache and trigeminal neuralgia. A non-prescription capsaicin cream called Zostrix is available to relieve pain and swelling associated with post-herpetic neuralgia.

CHERRY

Cherries are a sweet fruit that have been used in folk medicine to treat arthritis, bladder infections, epilepsy, gallstones, gout, kidney stones and rheumatisms. The use of cherry juice to treat gout was popularized in the 1950's. The consumption of cherry juice was believed to flush the kidneys of uric acid and reduce the joint pains associated with gout. Cherries have a mild diuretic effect that increases urine output in the kidneys. Cherries are rich in bioflavonoids that help to strengthen blood vessel walls and reduce inflammation. Cherries also contain chemicals that have potent antibiotic effects. Unsweetened cherry juice may help to fight common infections due to bacteria and viruses. Cherries can also inhibit tooth decay by preventing bacteria in the mouth from causing plaque formation. Cherries are good for treating obesity and aiding in weight loss. They are sweet, contain no fat or cholesterol and are low in calories.

CRANBERRY

Cranberries have been used in folk medicine to treat kidney stones, bladder problems and urinary tract infections. Cranberries contain a high amount of benzoic acid and other related compounds that the body metabolizes into hippuric acid. Hippuric acid prevents bacteria from sticking to the walls of the bladder, urethra and ureters. Hippuric acid has antibiotic effects against E. coli, the bacteria resposible for 85% of urinary tract infections. A high fluid intake should accompany intake of cranberries so that the fluid can flush the urinary tract of bacteria. A large consumption of unsweetened cranberry juice has been scientifically proven to decrease the occurence and duration of bladder and urinary tract infections. Cranberries may be useful in treating other common bacteria and viral infections throughout the body. Cranberries may be effective in breaking up calcium type kidney stones. Cranberries are also rich in bioflavonoids that help to strengthen blood vessel walls and reduce inflammation.

DATE

Dates and their close cousins, figs, are sweet tasting fruits that have been widely consumed since biblical times. They have been used in folk medicine to treat anemia, constipation, indigestion and to rid the body of parasites and worms. Dates contain a large amount of fiber and pectin. The high fiber content of this fruit makes it useful in treating constipation. Dates also have a natural laxative effect. They may be useful in treating heartburn and reducing stomach acid. Dates are a highly alkaline food that helps to neutralize acid in the stomach. Dates also contain natural enzymes called ficins that aid in digestion. Other chemicals in dates destroy parasites and worms in the digestive system. Dates also help to fight cancer. They contain a high amount of a chemical called benzaldehyde. Benzaldehyde interferes with the breakdown sugar and fermentation within cancer cells. Benzaldehye also prevents the break-down and increases the lifespan of red blood cells. Dates are also a good source of potassium.

GARLIC

Garlic is a strong scented perennial plant with long, flat and firm leaves that is widely used as a culinary spice. Garlic has been used in folk medicine for thousands of years by various cultures to treat colds, respiratory infections, whooping cough, bronchitis, toothache, earache and many other conditions too numerous to list here. Active ingredients isolated in garlic include allicin and other sulfur containing compounds at 0.1 to 0.5% of the dry weight of the bulb. Garlic has broad spectrum antibiotic activity against bacteria, viruses, fungi and parasites. Garlic decreases atherosclerosis in arteries, thins the blood, inhibits clot formation, decreases blood cholesterol levels and decreases blood pressure. It also has some anti-tumor effects. Garlic may be used as a broad spectrum antibiotic to treat common infections of the digestive system, urinary tract, respiratory system and the ears. Garlic may be used to help lower high blood pressure and high cholesterol. It can also be used to inhibit blood clot formation in individuals with atherosclerosis, heart disease or strokes.

GINGER

Ginger is a perennial plant that grows up to 1 meter in height and is native to southern Asia and the tropics including India, China, Jamaica, Haiti and Nigeria. The root is highly aromatic and is the source of dried powdered spice widely used as to flavor food and drink. Ginger root has been used for thousands of years in the Orient. It has been used in folk medicine to treat indigestion, diarrhea, nausea, toothache, poisoning, snakebite and rheumatisms. It also induces sweating, relieves intestinal gas and stimulates the appetite. Volatile oils are the active ingredients believed to be responsible for the therapeutic effects of this plant. The concentration of volatile oils ranges between 0.25 and 3.5% of the dry weight of the root. The volatile oils inhibit the growth of various bacteria and parasites, reduces fever, decreases pain, decreases coughs, decreases nausea and improves digestion. It also has immune stimulating effects, reduces blood cholesterol and has some anti-cancer effects. Ginger has been scientifically proven to reduce the symptoms of motion sickness, spinning sensation and dizziness. Ginger also has been proven to help relax stomach upset, indigestion and nausea. Ginger is relatively non-toxic and few side effects have been reported. However, it may cause stomach upset and in large doses can cause nervous system and heart beat irregularities.

GRAPEFRUIT

Grapefruit has been used in folk medicine to treat bladder problems, constipation, fungal infections, insomnia, kidney stones, nervousness, scurvy, skin infection and sore throats. Grapefruit has been widely used to help treat obesity and aid in weight loss. The grapefruit diet popularized the use of this fruit. Grapefruit contains no cholesterol, is low in sodium and high in vitamin C. Like all citrus fruits, grapefruit is rich in vitamin C. One grapefruit contains 100% the recommended daily requirement of vitamin C. Vitamin C is a potent antioxidant that helps to prevent free radical damage to the body. The antioxidant effects of grapefruit make this fruit beneficial in preventing the development of cancer. One medium-sized grapefruit contains about 3.0 grams of fiber. The high fiber content of this fruit makes it useful in lowering cholesterol levels. The cholesterol reducing capacity of grapefruit has been compared to the drug cholestyramine which is widely prescribed for high cholesterol. Grapefruit helps to reverse hardening of the arteries. A chemical in grapefruit called galacturonic acid helps to prevent plaque formation inside arteries. Grapefruit is also very good in lowering blood pressure. Grapefruit is a mild diuretic that increases urine output in the kidneys. Grapefruit helps to flush toxins from the body. It is also very good in promoting weight loss.

HONEY

Honey has been used in folk medicine for thousands of years. The Egyptians, Greeks and Romans used honey to cure a wide variety of ailments. Honey was used as a topical antiseptic to prevent wounds from getting infected. Honey contains a large amount of simple carbohydrates mainly as sucrose. Unlike refined sugar, honey also contains resins, aromatic oils, fats, and small amounts of vitamins and minerals. The resins and oils have potent anti-microbial effects against bacteria, viruses and fungi. The resins and oils are incorporated into the honey to prevent microbes from infecting the bee hives. The topical application of honey works remarkably well in preventing cuts and wounds from getting infected and accelerating the healing time. Honey provides a strong barrier over cuts and wounds and the oils, keeps germs out, destroys microbes and stimulates the healing process. Honey works as well as other topical antibiotic ointments such as polysporin and neosporin. Honey is also good in treating infectious diarrhea. The strong antibiotic effects kills microbes responsible for causing diarrhea. Honey is useful in treating anxiety, nervousness and insomnia. Honey exerts a calming effect on the nervous system. Honey stimulates production of a chemical in the brain called serotonin that relaxes the nervous system. A teaspoon of honey before bedtime may help you sleep better. A teaspoon of honey can help cure hiccups. Honey is also useful in treating colds and sore throats. It is often added to medicines to make them taste better. Honey not only helps to kill bacteria and viruses but also helps to reduce irritated and painful throats. Regular consumption of honey may be useful in treating allergies, asthma and hayfever. Honey contains small amounts of plant pollens. The small amount of pollens may help to desensitize the body to the airborne inhalents and build up the immune system.

LEMON

Lemons have been used in folk medicine to treat asthma, colds, coughs, hiccups, indigestion, skin rashes and sore throats. Lemons are a good source of vitamin C and bioflavonoids. They have been consumed to cure vitamin C deficiency or scurvy by many English sailors. The high vitamin C content of this fruit makes it beneficial in preventing cancer. Lemons are a good source of dietary fiber. A medium-sized lemon contains 2.4 grams of fiber. The high fiber content of this fruit makes it useful in lowering cholesterol and blood pressure. Lemon juice contains aromatic oils that account for the distinct odour of this fruit. Lemon oil has strong antimicrobial effects against bacteria, viruses and fungi. The topical application of lemon juice helps to fight common skin infections. The sour taste of lemons helps to stimulate digestive juices in the stomach. A small amount of lemon juice before meal time primes the stomach and improves digestion. Lemons also help to bind toxins in the digestive system before they are absorbed into general circulation.

LICORICE

Licorice is a perennial plant that grows between 1 to 2 meters in height and is native to Asia, Europe, parts of the Middle East and naturalized to North America. Roots and rhizomes of this plamt have been used for centuries as a condiment to flavor candies and tobacco. Licorice has been used in folk medicine to treat a variety of illness including asthma, bronchitis, diabetes, inflammation, indigestion and constipation. Triterpenoid glycosides are the active ingredients and are believed to be responsible for the therapeutic effects of this plant. The triterpenoid content of licorice ranges between 1 to 27% of the dry weight of the root. The average triterpenoid content ranges between 7 and 15%. The main triterpenoid compound in licorice is glycyrrhizin. Glycyrrhizin is responsible for the sweetness of licorice root and is 50 to 100 times sweeter than sugar. Licorice supports and stimulates the adrenal gland function, helps the body to reduce inflammation and respond to stress. Licorice coats the stomach and intestines and prevents inflammation of the digestive system. Licorice is a mild expectorant and helps to break up throat and chest congestion. Glycyrrhizin has estrogenic activity and may be useful in treating female disorders. Licorice may be beneficial in treating indigestion, inflammation of the digestive system, irritable bowel syndrome, constipation and peptic ulcers. Licorice may be useful in treating premenstrual syndrome, menstrual irregularities and menopause. High doses of licorice for prolonged periods of time may cause a condition known as pseudo-aldosteronism, marked by electrolyte imbalance, swelling, edema and high blood pressure. Deglycyrrhizinated licorice or DGL preparations do not cause this condition.

OATS

Oats have been used in folk medicine to treat anxiety, constipation, heartburn, indigestion, insomnia, nervousness and ulcers. Oatmeal has been used as an aphrodisiac and to treat impotence in males. Oatmeal pastes and baths have been recommended for eczema, psoriasis, and atopic dermatitis. Green oats have been used successfully in India to help cure nicotine and opium addiction. Oats are a rich source of dietary fiber. One half cup of rolled oats contains 3.6 grams of fiber. The high fiber content of oats makes this food useful in decreasing elevated blood cholesterol, high blood pressure and blood sugar irregularities. Soluble fiber in oats helps to decrease LDL or "bad" cholesterol and increase HDL or "good" cholesterol. Fiber in oats increases stool bulk and helps to cure constipation. Oats also have a natural laxative effect. Complex sugars in oats are highly mucilaginous. When oats are mixed with water they form a slimy paste that helps to decrease inflammation and itching on the skin. Oat paste and baths have been used to reduce symptoms associated with poison ivy. Oats are a rich source of protein. One half cup of oats contains 5.7 grams of protein. Oats also contain protease inhibitors that help to fight cancer

OLIVE OIL

Olive oil was first used by Egyptians for thousands of years. In more recent times olive oil has been widely used by Europeans. Olive oil was used in folk medicine to treat constipation, gallstones, liver congestion and peptic ulcers. Like all fats and oils, olive oil is high in calories. One gram of olive oil produces 9 calories of energy. However, olive oil is a mono-unsaturated fat and it has potent health benefits. Olive oil has been scientifically proven to decrease cholesterol levels. Olive oil helps to lower the total cholesterol level, decrease LDL or "bad" cholesterol and increase HDL or good cholesterol. Cultures that have the highest intake of olive oil include Italians and Greeks. They also have one of the lowest incidence of cardiovascular disease in developed countries. Olive oil helps to thin the blood, decrease blood clotting and decrease hardening of the arteries. Olive oil may be decrease the occurence of heart attacks, strokes and intermittent claudication. Olive oil may also help to lower high blood pressure. Olive oil also helps to contract the gall bladder and expel bile from the bile duct into the small intestine.

ONION

Onions have been widely used in folk medicine to treat bronchitis, chest congestion, colds, earaches, flus, heart problems, insomnia, kidney problems, intestinal infections, nasal congestion, nervousness, repiratory infections and skin infections. The distinctive odour of onions is due the high concentration of sulfur containing chemicals in this vegetable. Onions have been scientifically proven to lower total cholesterol and increase HDL or "good" cholesterol levels. Onions have strong anti-coagulant properties that help to thin the blood and prevent clot formation. They may be useful in treating heart attacks, strokes and intermittent claudication. They help to lower high blood pressure and help control blood sugar irregularities. Onions were once widely used to treat diabetes. The action of onions in lowering blood sugar levels has been compared to conventional oral hypoglycemic drugs. Onions have potent anti-microbial activity against bacteria, fungi and viruses. Onions are a natural expectorant that helps to break up mucous and phlegm in the throat, bronchi and lungs. Onions contain potent anti-cancer chemicals that help to fight cancer.

ORANGE

Oranges have been used in folk medicine to treat asthma, bronchitis, colds, coughs and fatigue. Oranges are one of the highest natural sources of vitamin C and bioflavonoids. One medium-sized orange contains 100% of the recommended dietary intake of vitamin C. Oranges have been used to treat vitamin C deficiency or scurvy in English sailors. The high vitamin C content of oranges helps to build and maintain strong connective tissue, strong gums and teeth and healthy bones. Oranges help to fight cancer. Oranges are a good source of dietary fiber. One medium-sized orange contains 2.6 grams of fiber. The high fiber content of oranges makes this fruit useful in decreasing blood cholesterol, blood pressure and blood sugar irregularities. Orange juice contains aromatic oils that account for the distinctive odour of this fruit. Orange oil has demonstrated strong anti-microbial activity against certain bacteria and viruses. Oranges are rich in fiber and water and low in calories. Oranges are a good food for individuals who want to lose weight. Oranges a rich in water and have a mild diuretic effect that helps to flush the kidneys and urinary tract. Oranges are also rich in citric acid. The citric acid content has an anticoagulant effect that helps to thin the blood and prevent clotting. Citric acid can also irritate the stomach in individuals with sensitive stomachs.

PEARS

Pears have been used in folk medicine to treat constipation, diarrhea, gallstones, indigestion and stomach problems. Pears are a rich source of dietary fiber. One medium-sized pear contains 4.2 grams of fiber. The high fiber content of pears makes this fruit useful in decreasing blood cholesterol levels, high blood pressure and blood sugar irregularities. Pears help to improve bowel regularity. They can be used can treat constipation or diarrhea. Pears are high in water content, low in calories and are a great fruit for individuals on calorie restricted diets.

PEAS

Peas are a member of the bean or legume family. Peas have been used in Indian and Tibetan folk medicine as a natural contraceptive. Peas are a good source of dietary fiber. One half cup of peas contains 2.8 grams of fiber. The high fiber content of this vegetable makes it useful in decreasing blood cholesterol, high blood pressure and blood sugar irregularities. Peas are a good source of protein. One half cup of peas contains 4.2 grams of protein. Certain proteins in peas called protease inhibitors help to prevent cancer especially stomach, intestinal and colon cancer. Peas contain a chemical m-xylohydroquinone that decreases sperm count in males by 50%. Peas also alter female hormone levels and inhibit conception in females by 50%. Peas have some antimicrobial effects against certain bacteria and viruses in the digestive system. Some studies show that peas can help prevent appendicitis. Peas also have a mild diuretic effect that helps to flush out the kidneys and urinary tract.

PRUNES

Prunes have been widely used in folk medicine to help move the bowels. Prunes have a potent natural laxative effect. Unlike conventional drug laxatives prunes are not addictive and have virtually no side effects. Prunes are a good source of dietary fiber. Three medium-sized prunes with the skin contain 3.0 grams of fiber. The high fiber content of prunes helps to increase stool bulk and improve constipation. The high fiber content of this fruit also helps to lower cholesterol levels, high blood pressure and correct blood sugar irregularities. The high fiber content of prunes only partly explains the laxative effects of this fruit. Prunes are also a rich source of magnesium. Magnesium helps intestinal muscles to relax and draws out water from the colon wall. The high magnesium content of prunes is believed to work like other conventional laxatives such as epsom salts and milk of magnesia. Prunes are a good source of potassium and bioflavonoids.

SOYBEAN

Soybeans have been a dietary staple of Asia for thousands of years. Soybeans have been made into a variety of food products including soybean flour, meal, paste, oil, milk, miso and tofu. Soy sauce is a popular liquid added to flavour foods. Miso is a fermented soybean paste that is used in foods and soups. Tofu is a solid curd-like substance added to foods as a meat substitute. Soybeans are a rich source of dietary fiber. One cup of cooked soybeans contains 9.0 grams of fiber. The high fiber content of this vegetable is useful in treating elevated blood cholesterol, high blood pressure and blood sugar irregularities. Soybeans help to decrease LDL or "bad" cholesterol and increase HDL or "good" cholesterol levels. Soybeans decrease hardening of the arteries and plaque formation. Soybeans help to improve sugar levels in diabetics, decreasing the dosage of oral hypoglycemic drugs or insulin. The high fiber content increases stool bulk, helps to improve bowel regularity and treat constipation. Soybeans are a rich source of protein. One cup of cooked soybeans contains 29.0 grams of protein. Soybean protein is reported to help prevent the development of gallstones. Soybeans are a rich source of vitamins and minerals. One cup of cooked soybeans contains 200 milligrams of calcium, 150 milligrams of magnesium, 900 milligrams of potassium and 9.0 milligrams of iron. Soybeans help to prevent the development of cancer. Soybeans have a mild estrogenic effect. They have reported to increase estrogen levels and improve menopausal symptoms in women. The increased estrogen levels can also produce a contraceptive effect.

SPINACH

The mythical cartoon sailor man Popeye popularized the use of spinach to increase energy and vitality. Spinach was used in folk medicine to treat anemia, bladder problems, constipation, indigestion, fatigue and kidney problems. Spinach is a rich source of vitamins and minerals including iron and potassium. The high iron content makes this vegetable useful in treating iron deficiency anemia. Unlike conventional iron supplements spinach is not constipating. Spinach is a good source of dietary fiber. One half cup of cooked spinach contains 1.7 grams of fiber. The high fiber content of spinach makes this vegetable useful in decreasing blood cholesterol levels. Spinach is a rich source of vitamin A and beta-carotene. One half cup of cooked spinach contains over 100% the recommended dietary intake of vitamin A. Vitamin A and beta-carotene are potent antioxidants that help to prevent cancer. The green color of this vegetable is due to its high chlorophyll content. Both beta-carotene and chlorophyll are potent cancer fighters. Chlorophyll is a natural deodorant and chelator of toxins in the body. Spinach contains a small amount of chemicals called goitrogens that can inhibit thyroid gland activity. Large quantities of raw spinach can interfere with the production of thyroid hormone. Cooking spinach inactivates these goitrogens.

SQUASH AND PUMPKIN

Squash and pumpkin have been used throughout the world to help destroy intestinal parasites and worms. Oils in the seeds have potent anti-parasitic and anti-worm effects. Squash and pumpkin seeds have been recommended for prostate problems in men. These seeds are a rich source of zinc. The high zinc content can help benefit the prostate gland. Squash and pumpkin are a good source of dietary fiber. One cup of squash contains 2.4 grams of fiber. One cup of pumpkin contains 3.2 grams of fiber. The high fiber content of these vegetables makes them useful in treating elevated blood cholesterol, high blood pressure and blood sugar irregularities. They are also useful in treating constipation and have a natural laxative effect. The orange color of these vegetables is due to the high concentration of carotenoids including beta-carotene and vitamin C. These vitamins help to prevent cancer.

TOMATOES

Tomatoes are considered to be a fruit and not a vegetable. Tomatoes have been used in folk medicine to treat constipation, indigestion, and kidney problems. Tomatoes were once considered to be an aphrodisiac. Raw tomatoes are considered an alkaline food while cooked tomatoes are considered a highly acidic food. Tomatoes and other members of the Nightshade family have been reported to aggravate arthritis. While this is yet to be scientifically proven many people swear that a large consumption of this fruit can make joint pains worse. The acidic tendency of this fruit can irritate the stomach and possibly irritate joints. Tomatoes are a good source of vitamin A and vitamin C. These antioxidants help to prevent cancer. Tomatoes are also a good source of electrolytes including sodium and potassium. Tomato juice has been used to restore electrolyte balance in individuals with diarrhea. Tomatoes can help to prevent intestinal infections and appendicitis.

TUMERIC

Tumeric or curcumin is a perennial herb of the ginger family that is widely used as a culinary spice in Asia, India, Indonesia and other tropical countries. The root of this herb has been ground up to make a pungent spice. Tumeric is a major ingredient of curry powder and is also used in prepared mustard. Tumeric has been used in folk medicine to treat abdominal gas, arthritis, indigestion, liver problems, menstrual irregularities, pain and toothache. Tumeric has potent anti-inflammatory and anti-arthritic activity and is useful in treating rheumatoid arthritis, osteoarthritis and other disorders with chronic pain and inflammation. Tumeric is useful in treating atherosclerosis, elevated blood cholesterol, intermitent claudication, thrombosis and strokes. Tumeric helps to lower total cholesterol, decrease blood clotting and dilates blood vessels. Tumeric is useful in treating liver and gall bladder disorders. Tumeric helps to prevent damage to liver cell, increases bile production and cause the gall bladder to expel its contents into the digestive system. Tumeric also helps to enhance digestion. Tumeric may also help to prevent certain types of cancer.

YOGURT

Yogurt is a fermented dairy product that has been used by cultures throughout the world for hundreds of years. Yogurt has been used in folk medicine to treat all digestive complaints including abdominal bloating, colitis, constipation, diarrhea, flatulence, indigestion and stomach ulcers. Yogurt has been applied topically to rejuvenate the skin. Yogurt has been reported to increase lifespan and promote longevity. Yogurt is made from the action of lactobacillus bacteria on whole milk. The sharp taste of this food is due to fermentation of milk sugar. Lactobacilli bacteria digest milk sugar producing natural acids including lactic acid. However, not all milk sugar is fermented by the bacteria. Yogurt does contain some lactose and may produce symptoms in lactose intolerant individuals. Lactobacilli bacteria are a part of the normal flora of the human digestive system. They help to maintain a healthy digestive system and immune system. As a part of the normal flora they inhibit the growth of other bacteria and fungi. Lactobacilli produce a number of natural antibiotics including acidolin, acidophilin and hydrogen peroxide. Indiscriminate use of antibiotics has lead to widespread yeast infection. Lactobacilli have a strong reputation for fighting yeast infection including oral candida, intestinal candida and vaginal yeast infection. Yogurt helps to restore and maintain normal balance of bacteria in the digestive system. Yogurt helps to treat oral infections and canker sores. Yogurt helps to decrease heartburn and reduce stomach acidity. Yogurt helps to heal stomach and duodenal ulcers. Yogurt is very useful in treating infectious diarrhea. Yogurt helps to destroy "bad" bacteria and restore the normal "good" bacteria. Yogurt contains chemicals that help to prevent cancer especially mouth, stomach, intestinal and colon cancer. Yogurt is a good source of protein. One cup of plain yogurt contains 12.0 grams of protein. Yogurt is a dairy product and it does contain a small amount of cholesterol. However, yogurt does help to raise HDL or "good" cholesterol. Yogurt is a rich source of calcium and potassium. One cup of plain yogurt contains 425 milligrams of calcium and 540 milligrams of potassium.

PART III

Achieving Unlimited Health

16

Blood Chemistry

Blood is the fluid that circulates through the heart, arteries, capillaries and veins. Blood is the chief method of transport for many chemicals of the body and for oxygen from the lungs. It transports nutritive substances and metabolites to the cells of the body and removes waste products to the kidneys and the other organs of excretion. It has an essential role in the maintenance of fluid balance. In an emergency, cells and proteins carried in the blood are brought to the point of infection, or blood clotting substances are carried to a break in a blood vessel. The blood is the chief method of transport for hormones produced in glands. Blood helps to regulate body temperature by carrying excess heat from the interior to the exterior of the body. Blood vessels just under the surface of the skin dilate to help dissipate heat to the surrounding air.

Blood consists of two main different constituents: blood cells including red blood cells and white blood cells and plasma or the liquid portion of blood. Red blood cells compromise about 43% of the entire volume of the blood. White blood cells usually compromise less than 2% of the entire blood volume. Plasma or the fluid portion of the blood compromises the remaining 55% of blood volume. Plasma contains of 92% water, 7% proteins and less than 1% inorganic salts, organic substances other than proteins, dissolved gases, hormones, antibodies, enzymes, electrolytes, minerals and vitamins. Plasma contains many other chemicals that provide invaluable information about the internal state of the health of an individual. Biochemical tests can be performed on the plasma to alert the patient and physician to potentially dangerous levels of blood constituents that could lead to more serious conditions. Biochemical tests can also help aid in the diagnosis of a particular condition of the patient and assess the patient's status by establishing a baseline of normal levels for each individual. Blood chemistry values vary considerably from individual and individual. Particular blood chemistry values are as unique to one person as their own fingerprint.

Before beginning the diet program I usually recommend that all patients have a fasting blood chemistry test. The test is a relatively inexpensive blood test that offers considerable insight into the internal state of the blood and organs of an individual. The test must be fasting twelve hours to obtain true, accurate values. That means that you shouldn't eat or drink fluids, except water, for twelve hours. This is a relatively simple procedure. You shouldn't eat or drink fluids, except water, after supper in the evening, until the next morning when you go to have your blood drawn.

The blood chemistry profile is meant to analyze six important blood values that determine the internal state of health of an individual. The six profiles are cholesterol, HDL cholesterol, LDL cholesterol, glucose, triglycerides and uric acid. Abnormal values of these values are very accurate indicators of a poor internal state of health of an individual. These values are also important in predicting the onset of different diseases including atherosclerosis, cardiovascular disease, diabetes, gout, heart disease, hypoglycemia, kidney disease and liver problems. This blood chemistry profile can be done by simply asking your doctor to order the particular tests requested. If the doctor is reluctant to order these tests then you can approach the laboratory directly or approach another doctor.

Cholesterol

Cholesterol is a simple steroid molecule found in animal fats and oils. Fruits and vegetables contain no cholesterol. Blood cholesterol level is the single most significant indicator of atherosclerosis or hardening of the arteries. However, cholesterol is not as bad as it is made out to be. Cholesterol is essential for life. Cholesterol is a fatty, waxlike material that has many vital functions in the human body. It is used to form many hormones in the body, makes vitamin D, forms an insulating sheath around nerves, forms protective coverings around many body organs and combines with bile to aid in the digestion of fats. The liver manufactures enough cholesterol for the body's needs. Seventy-five percent of the cholesterol in the average person's body is manufactured by the liver. Only 25% of the cholesterol in the average person's body is from foods we eat. The body can dispose of most extra cholesterol, but not all of it. Extra cholesterol obtained from diet builds up in the body. As cholesterol levels in the blood rise, cholesterol begins to be deposited inside the lumen or opening of arteries throughout the body. As cholesterol deposits build up inside arteries the flow of blood as restricted. Atherosclerosis or hardening of the arteries occurs. If cholesterol deposits build up unrestricted then the entire blood flow through a segment of an artery can be cut off. Serious consquences occur when this happens. To avoid this we need to be careful about the amount of cholesterol we eat each day.

The average North American consumes between 400 and 500 milligrams of cholesterol per day. This amount of cholesterol is too much. The American Heart Association recommends the average daily cholesterol intake should be between 100 and 300 mg per day. I usually recommend that the average daily cholesterol intake be between 100 and 200 mg per day. One medium-sized egg contains approximately 250 mg per day. Therefore, 1 egg per day would provide more than enough cholesterol to meet the body's entire daily requirement. To most people a low cholesterol diet means simply avoiding eggs and organs meats. However, we should remind ourselves that all animal products and their derivatives contain variable amounts of cholesterol. This means that all meat, chicken, fish, milk, cheese, ice cream, yogurt and other dairy products contain high amounts of cholesterol. We should also be wary of vegetable oils. Even though vegetable oils contain no cholesterol they are high in unsaturated fats. One gram of vegetable fat can raise cholesterol by one milligram. Therefore a diet high in unsaturated fats can raise blood cholesterol considerably. Total blood cholesterol level should be less than 5.2 mmol/liter or 200 mg/dl. A total blood cholesterol level greater than this upper limit is associated with increased risk of atherosclerosis. I like to see total blood cholesterol level less than 4.7 mmol/liter or 180 mg/dl for optimal health.

HDL Cholesterol

Like all fats and oils cholesterol doesn't mix well with water. The major ingredient in blood is water. To circumvent this problem of having cholesterol in blood the body use protein molecules to attach to cholesterol. Together the cholesterol and protein molecules form complex molecules called lipoproteins. There are several different types of lipoproteins in the blood.

HDL cholesterol called high density lipoprotein is commonly referred to as "good" cholesterol. Blood HDL levels are inversely associated the development of atherosclerosis. This means the higher the HDL level in your blood the less risk you have of having a cardiovascular accident. HDL transports cholesterol and fats from the arteries and takes it back to the liver where it can be disposed of. A HDL cholesterol count greater than 1.2 mmol/liter or 45 mg/dl for men and 1.4 mmol/liter or 55 mg/dl for women is beneficial.

Many native cultures throughout the world have very low HDL cholesterol levels and have a remarkably low incidence of cardiovascular problems. However, their overall cholesterol levels are also very low, usually less than 3.9 mmol/liter or 150 mg/dl.

LDL Cholesterol

LDL cholesterol called low density lipoprotein is commonly referred to as "bad" cholesterol. LDL cholesterol transports cholesterol and fats from the liver and digestive system to the arteries where it can be deposited and form atherosclerotic plaques. A LDL cholesterol count greater than 3.4 mmol/liter or 130 mg/dl is associated with the increased risk of cardiovascular problems.

Glucose

Glucose is the main source of energy for the cells of the body. During digestion carbohydrates are broken down into simple sugars in the digestive system. The simple carbohydrates or sugars are absorbed into the bloodstream and are carried to all cells of the body. The simple sugars enter the cells and are further broken down inside cells to produce energy.

Glucose is the simplest and most common sugar that is utalized by the body. Blood sugar levels are usually tightly regulated by the body. High blood sugar levels are associated with diabetes mellitus. Low blood sugar levels are associated with hypoglycemia or low blood sugar. Fasting blood sugar levels normally range between 3.8 and 6.7 mmol/liter or 70 and 120 mg/dl. An abnormally high fasting sugar reading is suggestive of diabetes and further tests may be warranted to determine the exact cause of this. An abnormally low fasting blood sugar reading is suggestive of hypoglycemia and further blood tests may be warranted to determine the cause of this. I usually recommend that fasting blood sugar levels should be less than 5.8 mmol/liter or 105 mg/dl for optimal health.

Triglycerides

Triglycerides are a simple form of fat that circulates in the blood. Triglycerides are a neutral fat that is the usual transport and storage form of fatty acids in the blood and body. Triglycerides consists of three molecules of fatty acids bound with one molecule of glycerol. Elevated blood triglyceride levels are now considered as important as high cholesterol in the development of atherosclerosis and heart disease. High levels of triglycerides are associated with obesity and atherosclerosis. One gram of fat can raise cholesterol levels by one milligram. The normal range for blood triglycerides is 0.23 to 1.8 mmol/liter or 20 to 160 mg/dl. I usually recommend fasting blood triglyceride level to be 1.4 mmol/liter or 120 mg/dl or less for optimal health.

Uric Acid

Uric acid is the end product of amino acid metabolism in the human body. Uric ucid is manufactured from the breakdown of a class of compounds called purines. Purines are found in high amounts in meats, especially organ meats, chicken, fish, shellfish, butter, cheese, eggs, sweet breads and pastries and other refined foods, beans, legumes and peas.

Uric acid is excreted in the urine in amounts of less than 1 gram per day. The presence of high concentration of uric acid in the blood is significant in the diagnosis of gout. The acute form of gout usually begins suddenly, without warning. 70% of attacks involve the big toe of the foot, although other joints including the foot, ankle, knee, wrist and elbow may be involved. Throbbing, crushing and excruciating pain of the affected joints occurs. Individuals with gout may be bedridden or have difficulty walking due to the pain. Swelling, tenderness of the overlying skin results. The skin may be a hot, shiny dusky red or purple color. Slight fever, rapid heart beat, headache, chills and malaise can be associated with gout.

With gout there is an excess of uric acid in the blood. Uric acid in the blood can form salts called urates that can form crystalline deposits in the kidneys and urinary system, joints and other tissues. High levels of uric acid in the blood can overload the kidneys. Normally uric acid is filtered and excreted by the kidneys in the urine. High levels or uric acid can overwhelm the kidneys and impair their ability to effectively excrete uric acid. As a result uric acid levels back up in the blood. Uric acid can form salts in the blood called urates. The uric acid salts form crystalline deposits in the kidneys, urinary tracts joints and other tissues throughout the body.

The normal range for blood uric acid levels is 0.15 to 0.50 mmol/liter or 2.5 to 8.0 mg/dl. I usually recommend that all fasting blood uric acid levels be less than 0.36 mmol/liter or 6.0 mg/dl for optimal health.

17

Unlimited Diet and Nutrition

Diet, nutrition and the therapeutic use of foods have always been a cornerstone of naturopathic medicine. A growing body of scientific knowledge in this area is reflected by the numerous professional journals of nutrition and dietary sciences. Many medical conditions can be treated as effectively with foods and nutritional supplements as they can be by any other means, but with fewer complications and side effects. Naturopathic physicians receive over 200 hours of training in diet and clinical nutrition. In contrast, most medical doctors receive fewer than 20 hours of education. Natural food, good nutrition and diet therapy are required for achieving optimal health.

Dieting and losing weight are big business in North America. Walk into a bookstore and browse at the diet section. There are hundreds of different books on diet. There are The Candida Diet, Diabetic Diet, Eat to Win, Fit for Life, The Grapefruit Diet, The Hollywood Diet, The Hypoglycemic Diet, The Pritikin Diet, The Scaresdale Diet, The T-Diet and many other diets and diet books too numerous to list here. There are numerous diet centers and weight loss clinics. There is Jenny Craig, Nutri-System Weight Loss Centers, Physician Weight Loss Center and many other clinics too numerous to list here. I came to the conclusion that diets don't work after reviewing hundreds of different diet books. The information presented was often confusing, conflicting and contradictory. One diet says one thing while another diet says something totally opposite. I've actually stopped reading diet books because of this. The simple truth is that diet don't work. There is no magic diet or diet pill. Short term dieting to lose weight is ineffective. There really is only one effective diet. And that is a diet for life. Instead of dieting for two weeks or one month we should all develop proper dietary habits that we maintain throughout life.

Diet Is Individualistic

There is no one universal diet. It is impossible give perfect dietary information to one person. Each person's body type, makeup, requirements, likes, dislikes, allergies and sensitivities are unique. The diet of one culture, family or person may not be suitable for another culture, family or person. A vegetarian diet may not be suitable for one person, whereas a high meat diet may not be suitable for another person. Food sensitivities and food allergies are vary from one person to another. What one man can eat with impunity is another man's poison. Dietary advice and counselling should be highly individualistic.

10 Principles of a Healthy Diet

1. Eat only whole, pure, natural, unprocessed foods.
2. Avoid all processed and refined foods.
3. Eat a variety of foods, fresh fruits and vegetables.
4. Don't overeat and eat only when hungry.
5. Eat three meals per day.
6. Avoid eating when hurried or stressed.
7. Eat foods that are in season and native to your environment.
8. Chew your food thoroughly.
9. Eat raw foods before cooked foods.
10. Follow simple principles of food combining.

Water and Diet

Water is a rather simple chemical that is necessary for life. Water is a neutral, universal solvent. The human body is approximately 93% water. You can live without food for prolonged periods of time, but you can't live without water. Some animals and plants can live without water for days, but the human body was designed to consume water every day. Daily water requirement varies from person to person and from climate to climate. A person in a tropical climate who perspires easily will probably drink more water than a person in a cold climate who is trying to conserve water. The minimum recommended daily intake of water is the equivalent of 6 to 8 twelve ounce glasses per day. Pure, natural spring water is a good source of water. Spring water contains various minerals in addition to plain water. Flouridated water has been associated with certain cancers and bone disease. Distilled water has no natural minerals.

To Drink Or Not To Drink with Meals?

There is always controversy when it comes to the question of whether or not to drink water with meals. When you eat a meal you mix solid and semi-solid food in the stomach. The stomach and intestines produce enzymes to help digest the food. When you mix a little water or fluids with a meal it helps to liquify food and make digestion easier. However, if you consume large amounts of water or fluids with a meal you dilute the digestive juices too much. A large amount of fluids tends to dilute the enzymes in the stomach and make their job of digesting foods much harder. The stomach and intestines have to work twice as hard to digest the food. The key is to drink water in moderation when eating meals. One 12 ounce glass of water is recommended per meal. Do not drink ice cold water with meals. Ice cold water shocks the stomach and inhibits normal production of enzymes in the digestive system. It is better to drink room temperature or slightly cool water with meals.

Chew Thoroughly

Mastication is the process of chewing our food. The purpose of mastication is to break down large chunks of food into smaller chunks so that they can be digested in the stomach. Saliva contains enzymes that begin the digestive process. Saliva also helps to lubricate food to make swallowing easier. The tongue and mouth contain taste buds that allow us to taste our food. We are often reminded in our childhood to chew our food slowly and carefully. This simple rule also applies to adults. If you gobble your food, fail to chew carefully and eat on the run proper digestion is prevented. To ensure proper digestion it is important to chew your food slowly and thoroughly.

Food combining

Food combining means that foods should be eaten in certain, simple combinations to ensure optimal digestion and absorption. All foods can be classified as either acid or alkaline. Acid foods require acid enzymes to be broken down and absorbed in the digestive system. Alkaline foods require alkaline enzymes to be broken down and absorbed in the digestive system. Acid and alkaline foods don't mix well together and make digestion difficult. To ensure optimal digestion and absorption acid and alkaline foods should not be eaten together at the same meal.

Acid Ash/Alkaline Ash

After you burn wood in a fire the residue remaining is called ash. Ash is also the term used to describe the end products of digestion. All foods can be classified as acid or alkaline ash. Acid ash is used to describe acidic end products of digestion. Alkaline ash is used to describe alkaline end products of digestion. A diet high in fats and oils, protein, processed and refined foods, sugar and refined carbohydrates produces an acid ash. A diet high in whole grains and cereals, fresh fruits and vegetables produces an alkaline ash.

PH and High School Chemistry

PH is the term used to describe whether a solution is acid or alkaline. By definition, an acid is a substance that can give up a hydrogen ion. The positively charged hydrogen ion is considered the active constituent of all acids. A base is a substance that can accept a hydrogen ion. The more acidic a substance is the greater its concentration of hydrogen ions is and the greater its ability to give up hydrogen ions. All solutions can be described as either acid, neutral or alkaline. The degree to which a substance is acid or alkaline is measured on the pH scale. Chemists devised a simple scale from 1.0 to 14.0 to describe the degree of acidity or alkalinity. A pH of 7.0 is considered neutral. Any pH number below 7.0 is considered acidic. Any pH number above 7.0 is considered alkaline. A pH of 6.0 is considered slightly acidic. A pH of 5.0 is considered to be ten times more acidic than 6.0. A pH of 4.0 is considered to be a hundred times more acidic than 6.0. A pH of 8.0 is considered slightly alkaline. A pH of 9.0 is considered ten times more alkaline than 8.0. A pH of 10.0 is considered a hundred times more alkaline than 8.0.

Acid-Base Balance

The overall pH of the human body is slightly alkaline. The pH of the human body is between 7.35 to 7.45. The acid-base balance in the human body is tightly regulated. The body can tolerate and compensate for slight deviations in acidity and alkalinity. However, if the pH drops below 7.30 a potentially serious condition called acidosis occurs. If the pH goes higher than 7.50 then a state called alkalosis occurs. In either case the disturbance of acid-base balance is considered serious and could potentially be fatal.

Acid/Base Regulation

The acid-base balance in the human body is tightly regulated. Most of the body's metabolic processes produce acids as their end products. However, a somewhat more alkaline body fluid is required as a medium for vital cellular activities. Therefore, chemical exchanges of hydrogen must take place continuously in order to maintain a state of equilibrium. An optimal pH between 7.35 and 7.45 must be maintained. Otherwise, enzyme systems and other biochemical and metabolic activities will not function normally.

Shifts in pH in body fluids are controlled by three regulatory systems. Hydrogen ions, proteins and enzymes and the kidneys play an important role of acid/base balance. Chemicals in the blood help to buffer hydrogen ions. When there are a lot of acids in the blood there are a lot of hydrogen ions. The excess hydrogen ions attach to bicarbonate and other alkaline ions to form neutral chemicals that don't affect pH. Proteins and enzymes in the blood and body's fluids can help to maintain proper pH balance in the body. The kidneys play an important role in maintaining acid/base balance in the body. If the blood is acidic then it contains a large concentration of hydrogen ions and other acids. The excess hydrogen ions and acids can be filtered by the kidneys and excreted in urine. If the blood is alkaline then it contains a small concentration of acids. The kidneys can cause retention of hydrogen ions and acids and help to maintain proper pH balance. The skin also plays an important role in acid/base balance. Sweating helps to eliminate excess acids.

Measuring pH in the Body

Sometimes it is difficult to measure the overall pH of the body. The pH of other organs and tissues can be measured. The pH of the mouth should be between 7.0 and 7.5. The pH of the stomach should be between 2.0 and 6.0. The pH of the intestines should be between 6.0 and 7.0. The pH of the urine should be between 6.0 and 6.5. If the pH of the mouth is less than 7.0 or the pH of the urine is less than 6.0 then the body is considered acidic and a state of acidosis exists.

Acidosis

If the pH of the body goes lower than 7.30 a condition called acidosis results. Acidosis results from the accumulation of acid or depletion of the body's alkaline reserves in the blood and body tissue. As a result the concentration of hydrogen ions increases and consequently the body pH drops.

Chronic Disease

Most chronic diseases are acid forming in the human body. Arthritis is largely due to formation of acids in joints. Diabetes is associated with the formation ketoacids. Gout is a painful inflammation of joints, primarily the big toe, due to excessive accumulation of uric acid in joints. Cancer is a group of diseases characterized by rapid, uninhibited cell growth. All different types of cancer have the same biochemical characteristics. They primarily depend upon anaerobic metabolism for the energy. Anaerobic metabolism literally means metabolism without oxygen and is a rapid, quick way of producing energy. However, the byproducts of anaerobic metabolism are acid waste products. These acid waste products accumulate in the body and lead to a highly acidic human body. A diet rich in acid foods tends to produce an acid ash. As a result the body becomes acidic. A highly acidic body is considered toxic and can quickly lead to the development of chronic disease.

Metabolism

Metabolism is the term used to describe the sum total of all physical and chemical processes that occur within the human body. The goal of metabolism is build up and maintain the function of the human organism. Digestion, absorption and assimilation are vital parts of metabolism.

Anabolism/Catabolism

There are two phases of metabolism: anabolism and catabolism. Anabolism is a constructive phase. It is concerned with building up the human body. During this phase simple nutrients derived from digestion are used to make complex, living substances that are utalized by the body. Muscle, connective tissue, organs and other tissues are products of anabolism. Maintaining these vital tissues are anabolic processes. Catabolism is a destructive phase. It is concerned with the breakdown of complex substances to make simple chemicals that can be utalized by the body. During the process of catabolism energy is liberated. Energy is needed to maintain proper function of the human body. Most of the biochemical processes that occur inside the human body produce acids as their end products.

Acid Foods

All protein foods are acid forming. Protein foods are high in amino acids which are used by the body to make muscle, connective tissue and enzymes. Acid enzymes are required to digest protein foods. To digest protein the stomach produces large quantities of hydrochloric acid. The end products of protein digestion is an acid ash or residue.

Some fruits are acidic including lemons, limes and oranges. However, acid fruits tend to produce an alkaline ash. Cooked tomatoes are acidic. Soybeans and tofu derivatives are acidic. Refined and processed foods are highly acidic. Vinegar and pickled foods are acidic. Sugar and refined carbohydrates are slightly acidic. Chocolate, cookies, donuts and other sweets produce an acid ash. Coffee, tea and soft drinks are highly acidic. Deep fried foods including french fries are acidic. Refined and processed grains and cereals are acidic. White flour, pasta and other refined and processed grains are acidic. Gluten in wheat is acidic. An ideal diet should consist of only 20% acid foods.

Alkaline Foods

Almost all fresh fruits and vegetables are alkaline. Acid fruits including lemons, limes and oranges produce an alkaline ash. Raw tomatoes are alkaline, while cooked tomatoes are acidic. All non-starchy vegetables, whether cooked or raw, are alkaline. Whole, natural grains and cereals are alkaline. Brown rice, buckwheat, corn, flax, kamut, oats, millet, rye, spelt and whole wheat are alkaline. An ideal diet should consist of 80% alkaline foods.

Classification of Foods

All foods can be classified as acid or alkaline. There are acid fruit, sub-acid fruit, melons, sweet fruit, protein, non-starchy vegetables, grains and cereals and starchy vegetables.

Acid Fruit

Cranberries, grapefruit, kiwi, lemon, lime, orange, pineapple, pomegranate, rhubarb, tangerine, tomato

Sub-acid Fruit

Apple, apricots, blackberries, blueberries, cherries, grapes, huckleberries, peaches, pears, plums, raspberries, strawberries

Melons

Canteloupe, honeydew melon, muskmelon, watermelon

Sweet Fruit

Bananas, carob, currants, dates, figs, raisins and dried fruit

Protein

Meat including beef, lamb, organ meats, pork, veal, venison, wild game; poultry including chicken, duck, turkey; fish including bass, cod, halibut, red snapper, salmon, sole, trout,tuna; shellfish including clams, crab, lobster, oysters, prawns, shrimp; Dairy products including butter, buttermilk, cheese, milk, yogurt; Eggs; Nuts including almonds, brazil nuts, cashews, filberts, peanuts, peanut butter, walnuts

Non-starchy Vegetables

Alfalfa sprouts, artichokes, bamboo shoots, beets, bok choy, broccoli, brussel sprouts, cabbage, carrots, cauliflower, celery, chives, collards, cucumber, dandelion, egg plant, garlic, kale, leek, lettuce, mushrooms, mustard greens, okra, onion, parsley, peas, peppers, radishes, spinach, watercress

Grains and Cereals

Barley, flax, kamut, millet, oats, rice, rye, spelt, triticale, wheat

Starchy Vegetables

Beans, corn, lentils, parsnips, potatoes, pumpkin, squash, yams

Unlimited Diet

An ideal diet should consist 6 vegetables, 2 pieces of fruit, 1 serving of protein and 1 serving of starch each day. Ideally, 60% percent of foods should be raw and 40% of foods should be cooked. Eighty percent of foods should be alkaline and 20% of foods should be acidic. Care should be taken not to combine acid and alkaline foods at one meal. This means you should be careful when eating acid foods such as protein with alklaine foods such as fruit, grains and cereals and starchy vegetables. Non-starchy vegetables and fats and oils tend to be neutral and combine well with either acid or alkaline foods.

18

Menu Suggestions and Recipes

Breakfast

Breakfast is the most important meal of the day. The purpose of breakfast is to break the fast of the night and to supply the body with energy to meet the demands of the day. Carbohydrates are easy to digest foods that help break the fast of the previous night. Carbohydrates are also the best foods for supplying the body with energy. Therefore, breakfast should consist of simple and complex carbohydrates. Breakfast should include complex carbohydrates such as grains, cereals and starchy vegetables and simple carbohydrates such as fruit. Bacon and eggs are protein foods and are not good breakfast choices. They don't supply the body with energy, they take a long time to be digested and are not an appropriate breakfast food.

There should be seasonal variation in foods consumed. In winter when it is cold outside we should consume warming foods to help warm the body. Therefore, hot grains and cereals would be appropriate warming foods. In summer when it is cold outside we should consume cooling foods to help cool the body. Therefore, cold grains and cereals would be appropriate cooling foods. For optimal digestion we should restrict our breakfast to carbohydrates.

Lunch

Lunch is the intermediate meal of the day. The purpose of lunch is allow time to take a break from the work of the day and replenish the body with energy for the rest of the day. Carbohydrates are the best foods to supply the body with energy. Lunch should consist of complex carbohydrates, non-starchy vegetables and fats and oils. Lunch should include complex carbohydrates such as grains, cereals and starchy vegetables, non-starchy vegetables and fats and oils.

There should be seasonal variation in foods consumed. In winter when it is cold outside we should consume warming foods to help warm the body. Therefore, hot grains and cereals, cooked starchy vegetables and cooked non-starchy vegetables should be consumed. In summer when it is warm outside we should consume cooling foods to help cool the body. Cold grains and cereals, uncooked starchy vegetables and uncooked non-starchy vegetables should be consumed. Protein should not be consumed at lunch. Protein does not really supply the body with energy, takes a long time to digested and interferes with the breakdown of carbohydrates. For optimal digestion we should limit the consumption of protein at lunch.

Supper

Supper is the final meal of the day after the day's work has been completed. The purpose of supper is to allow time to relax from the day's activities and replenish material that has been expended through the day. When we work through the day we traditionally use our body and muscles. Muscle and other tissue breaks down from the heavy demands of the day. They need time to relax and repair themselves. Protein supplies the body with the raw materials to repair itself. Proteins are rich in amino acids that can be utalized by the body to repair muscle and other tissues. Therefore, protein should be the main source of food consumed at supper time. Supper should consist of protein, non-starch vegetables and fats and oils. Simple carbohydrates such as fruit and sugar should not be consumed at supper time. Complex carbohydrates may be occasionally consumed at supper time depending on the state of health of an individual and the desire to lose weight.

Protein takes a long time to be digested and absorbed. It takes at least six hours to break down and absorb animal protein. It takes about four hours to break down and absorb non-animal protein. Simple carbohydrates are the quickest and simplest foods to digest. It takes less than one hour to digest and absorb simple carbohydrates. When we consume a large meal of protein and other heavy foods it takes a long time to digest and absorb the nutrients. If we add dessert in the form of simple carbohydrates we complicate the digestive process. Simple carbohydrates are rich in sugar and don't have to wait long to be digested. However, on a full stomach of protein and other heavy foods simple carbohydrates have to wait around till all other foods are digested before they can be absorbed. They are prevented from passing through the digestive system by protein and other heavy foods. Simple carbohydrates can literally ferment in the stomach and digestive system as they wait around for the other foods to be digested. This can lead to many problems such as indigestion, gas, bloating, heartburn, flatulence and yeast infection. Therefore, simple carbohydrates should not be consumed at supper time. This means no dessert after dinner.

Theoretically, you would have to wait at least four to six hours after the protein has been digested before consuming simple carbohydrates. Adding complex carbohydrates at supper time is optional depending upon the state of health of the individual and the desire to lose weight. If you are in a poor state of health or you desire to lose weight do not consume complex carbohydrates at supper time. You should not consume grains, cereals and starchy vegetables at supper time. This means you should not have potatoes, corn, squash, rice, bread, pasta or other grains and cereals at supper time. Non-starchy vegetables and fats and oils may be consumed at supper time as desired. Supper should consist of an animal or non-animal protein source, non-starchy vegetables and fats and oils.

There should be seasonal variation in the types and state of foods consumed. In winter when it is cold outside we should consume hot meals consisting of cooked protein and cooked non-starchy vegetables. In summer when it warm outside we should cooler meals consisting of cold or cooked protein and un-cooked starchy vegetables. In summer we should consume more salads and other cooling vegetables at supper.

Snacks

Snacks are allowed throughout the day. They are especially necessary for individuals that have blood sugar irregularities such as hypoglycemia or low blood sugar. You can have a mid-morning snack between breakfast and lunch, an afternoon snack between lunch and supper or an evening snack after dinner. There are no restrictions in the amount of times you can snack during the day. What is important is the type of foods you consume at snack time. You should follow the simple principles of food combining. Don't mix acid and alkaline foods when snacking. You should restrict consumption of simple carbohydrates close to supper time. Remember protein and other heavy foods to a long time to be digested. If you consume simple carbohydrates while you are digesting protein you can encounter indigestion, gas and bloating. To expediate the digestive process don't consume proteins with carbohydrates at snack time. Non-starchy vegetables and fats and oils tend to be relatively neutral and can be consumed with either protein or carbohydrates.

Breakfast Suggestions

Oatbran muffins, oatmeal biscuits, hearth bread, hearth muffins, corn bread, apple bran muffins, fruit cocktail, almond or cashew milk, atvar, hot lemon drink, sunflower carob milk, orange-banana frappe, super bran muffins, granola, buttermilk pancakes, millet, rolled oats, cream of wheat, muesli, immune support breakfast, oatmeal pancakes.

Lunch Suggestions

Apricot rice, oriental rice, pasta primavera, rice casserole, vegetarian pasta, spanish rice, stirfry, vegetarian chow mein, vegetarian chili, bean salad, ceasar salad, cole slaw, greek salad, macaroni salad, potato salad, tabouli, waldorf salad, borscht, carrot soup, cauliflower soup, gazpacho soup, ministrone soup, miso soup, onion soup, pea soup, potato leek soup, tomato soup, vegetable soup, vegetable stew, blue cheese dressing, catsup, chili sauce, creamy herb dressing, ginger sauce, honey mustard dressing, horseradish dressing, imitation sour cream, marinara sauce, oil and vinegar dressing, oriental dressing, salsa, tahini, teriyaki marinade, tofu mayonnaise, oatmeal muffins, oatmeal biscuits, corn bread, hearth bread, hearth muffins, millet, super bran muffins, beets in orange sauce, eggplant parmesan, garlic stirfry vegetables, honey and lemon carrots and apples, oriental broccoli, roasted garlic, sauteed carrots, vegetarian stirfry, zucchini cutlets.

Dinner Suggestions

Baked salmon, meat loaf, ratatouille, almond chicken, apricot giner chicken cajun cod, curried chicken, ginger fish, halibut with tarragon, hot and spicy red snapper, lemon chicken, oriental chicken salad, tuna salad, acorn squash, beets in orange sauce, eggplant parmesan, garden stirfry vegetables, honey and lemon carrots with apples, mashed potatoes, oriental broccoli, potato skins, roasted garlic, sauteed carrots, scalloped potatoes, vegetarian stirfry, zucchini cutlets, ceasar salad, cole slaw, greek salad, waldorf salad, borscht, carrot soup, cauliflower soup, cold cucumber soup, gazpacho soup, ministrone soup, miso soup, onion soup, pea soup, tomato soup, vegetable soup, vegetable stew, blue cheese dressing, catsup, chili sauce, creamy herb dressing, ginger sauce, honey mustard dressing, horseradish dressing, imitation sour cream, marinara sauce, oil and vinegar dressing, oriental salad, salsa, tahini, teriyaki marinade, tofu mayonnaise, almond or cashew milk, sunflower carob milk.

Snacks

Antipasto, fruit platter, guacamole, homemade yogurt, hummus, mexican bean dip, salmon pate, salsa, trail mix, tzatsiki, vegetable platter, peach fizz, pineapple, grapefruit fizz, strawberry smoothie, yogurt fruit drink, honey nut bread, carrot cake, chutney, banana mousse, tapioca pudding, energy bars, fruit cocktail, fruit flan, oatbran muffins, oatmeal biscuits, hearth bread, hearth muffins, corn bread, apple bran muffins, super bran muffins, raisin bran muffins.

Sample One Week Menu

DAY 1

Breakfast - Hot lemon drink, rolled oats, unsweetened fruit.

Lunch - Vegetarian stirfry, garden salad and vegetable soup.

Snack - Fruit or vegetable, honey nut bread or oatbran muffin.

Dinner - Lemon chicken, oriental chicken salad, oriental broccoli.

DAY 2

Breakfast - Herbal tea, muesli, soy or nut milk, fruit cocktail.

Lunch - Ceasar salad, hearth bread, potato leek soup.

Snack - Homemade yogurt, fresh fruit in season, antipasto, tzatsiki.

Dinner - Meat loaf, garden salad, sauteed beets and carrots.

DAY 3

Breakfast - Hot lemon drink, oatmeal pancakes, unsweetened fruit.

Lunch - Pasta primavera, greek salad.

Snack - Carrot cake, muffin or fresh vegetables.

Dinner - Baked Halibut, garden stirfry vegetables, waldorf salad.

DAY 4

Breakfast - Herbal tea, immune support breakfast, unsweetened fruit.

Lunch - Oriental rice, vegetarian chow mein, teriyaki sauce.

Snack - Fresh fruit in season, fruit pudding, fruit cocktail.

Dinner - Zucchini cutlets, garden salad, mashed potatoes, beets.

DAY 5

Breakfast - Hot lemon drink, hearth toast, granola, soy or nut milk.

Lunch - Vegetarian chili, spanish rice, salsa.

Snack - Trail mix, mexican bean dip, hummus, vegetables.

Dinner - Almond chicken, vegetarian stirfry, acorn squash.

DAY 6

Breakfast - Herbal tea, atvar, muffin, fresh fruit in season.

Lunch - Vegetarian sandwich, onion soup, cole slaw.

Snack - Muffin, ginger snaps, energy bars.

Dinner - Ginger fish, garden salad, sauteed carrots.

DAY 7

Breakfast - Hot lemon drink, millet, unsweetened fruit.

Lunch - Spanish rice, tomato soup, bean salad.

Snack - Fresh fruit or vegetables in season.

Dinner - Ratatouille, ceasar or greek salad, cooked vegetables.

Appetizers and Snacks

ANTIPASTO

1 cup finely chopped cauliflower
1 cup ripe olives
1/4 cup finely chopped green olives
1/2 cup chopped pickled onions
1/4 cup vegetable oil
1 cup sliced mushrooms (canned)
1 small green pepper, finely chopped
2 cups catsup (see recipe)
1 cup sweet pickles, finely chopped, with juice saved
1/4 cup finely chopped red pepper (optional)
3 tablespoon sweet pickle juice
1 can water-packed light tuna

Mix cauliflower, olives, green olives, onions and vegetable oil in a large saucepan. Bring to boil over medium heat, then reduce heat and simmer for 10 minutes. Add mushrooms, green pepper, catsup, sweet pickles and red pepper. Bring to boil, then simmer for 10 more minutes. Stir often. Remove from heat and mixture cool. Stir in tuna. Serve cold with crackers, biscuits or bread. Makes 6 cups.

FRUIT PLATTER

1 cup canteloupe, sliced into chunks, wedges or balls
1 cup honeydew melon, sliced into chunks, wedges or slices
1 cup watermelon, sliced into chunks, wedges or slices
1 cup strawberries, whole or sliced
1 cup apples, cut into slices
1 cup papaya, sliced into chunks, wedges or balls
1 cup mango, sliced into chunks, wedges or balls
2 ripe kiwifruits, cut into slices

Use only fresh fruit in season. Prepare and arrange fruit on a large platter according to colour and variety. Serve chilled. Makes 12 servings.

GUACAMOLE

2 ripe medium avocadoes
2 teaspoons lemon juice
2 cloves crushes garlic
3 tablespoons chopped tomato
10 drops tabasco sauce
1/4 teaspoon salt (optional)
1/4 teaspoon fresh ground pepper (optional)

Peel, pit and cut avocadoes into chunks. In a small bowl mash avocadoes. Add seasonings and spices. Mix until well blended. Refrigerate until serving. Serve with vegetables and/or tortilla chips. Makes 4 servings.

HOMEMADE YOGURT

16 cups 2% milk
1 cup plain lowfat yogurt

Pour milk into a large pot. Bring to a rolling bowl on the stove. Reduce heat and simmer for 10 minutes. Remove from stove. Let cool to lukewarm temperature. Dilute 1 cup plain yogurt with 1 cup milk. Mix until well blended. Pour diluted mixture back into pot containing milk. Stir well until there are no lumps. Pour into jars or containers. Place on a towel away from draft in a warm environment. Cover lightly and let set for about 10 hours. Place in refrigerator and let cool. Wait 3 days and then you have yogurt. Makes 16 servings.

HUMMUS

1-16 ounce can chick peas
1/2 cup tahini
4 tablespoons lemon juice
1 clove chopped garlic
1/4 teaspoon salt (optional)
1/4 teaspoon ground cumin
1 tablespoon fresh chopped parsley

Drain liquid from chick peas. Combine all ingredients except parsley in a blender or food processor. Mix until well blended. Scrape from blender into a small wall. Refrigerate for at least 1 hour. Garnish with parsley. Makes 6 servings.

MEXICAN BEAN DIP

2-15 ounce cans of pinto beans
1 1/2 teaspoons ground cumin
1/4 teaspoon chili powder
2/3 teaspoon tabasco sauce
2 teaspoon lemon juice
1/4 teaspoon salt (optional)

Drain liquid from 1 can of pinto beans. Mix drained and undrained cans of pinto beans in a blender or food processor. Add seasonings. Mix until well blended. Scrape bean dip into a small bowl. Refrigerate until serving. Makes about 2 1/2 cups.

SALMON PATE

1 15 ounce can of salmon
2 tablespoons lemon juice
2 tablespoon chopped onion
1 tablespoon chopped fresh dill or 1 teaspoon dried dill
1 tablespoon plain gelatin
1/2 cup chopped onion
1/4 cup chopped parsley
1/2 teaspoon horseradish

Place salmon, lemon juice, onion and dill in a blender or food processor. Mix until well blended. In a medium saucepan dissolve gelatin with 2 tablespoon salmon mixture. Bring to a boil. Remove from heat and add gelatin to salmon. Stir in onions, parsley and horseradish. Refrigerate for 4 hours. Serve chilled. Makes 1 cup.

SALSA

2 14 ounce cans of tomatoes
1 mediums-sized green pepper, chopped into pieces
1/2 cup chopped onion
1 clove minced garlic
4 small jalapeno peppers, sliced

Put all ingredients in a blender or food processor. Mix until well blended. Pour ingredients into a saucepan. Bring to a boil. Simmer for 10 minutes. Cool and pour into a container. Serve as a sauce or dip. Makes 3 cups.

TRAIL MIX

1 cup peanuts (or other nuts if desired)
1 cup broken cashews
1/2 cup sunflower seeds
1 cup dried apricots cut into quarters
1/2 cup light raisins
1/2 cup dark raisins
1/2 cup dates

Mix all ingredients in a large bowl. Makes about 6 cups.

TZATSIKI

3 medium cucumbers
1 medium onion
2 cloves minced garlic
3 cups plain lowfat yogurt

Peel, remove the seeds and finely chop the cucumbers. Finely mince the onion and garlic. Combine all ingredients in a medium bowl. Mix until well blended. Refrigerate for at least 2 hours to allow ingredients to blend. Serve chilled. Makes about 4 cups.

VEGETABLE PLATTER

1 cup cauliflower, cut into florets
1 cup broccoli, cut into florets
1 medium-sized green pepper, cut into strips
1 1/2 cups carrots cut into sticks
1/2 cup radishes, sliced or cut into roses
3 celery stalks, cut into sticks
1/2 cup fresh, whole mushrooms
1/2 cup cherry tomatoes

Arrange all vegetables on a platter according to colour and variety. Place on or more dips or sauces desired. Serve chilled. Makes 12 servings.

Beverages

ALMOND OR CASHEW MILK

1 cup almonds or cashews
3 cups water
1 tablespoon honey
1 banana (optional)
3 tablespoons carob for carob milk

Mix 1 cup nuts with 1 cup water in a medium bowl. Add sweetener and carob to mixture. Blend all ingredients until creamy. Add remaining water until desired consistency. As a variation you can add 1/2 teaspoon of vanilla or maple flavourings. Add less water and frozen strawberries for a milkshake. Makes 4 cups.

ATVAR

2 cups dried prunes
1 cup dried apricots
1 cup dried peaches
1 cup dried apples and raisins

Wash fruit well. Place fruit in a large pot and cover with cold water. Soak overnight. Cook in the same water for 30 minutes. Sweeten with honey or natural sweeteners if desired. Serve cold or hot. Makes 5 cups.

HOT LEMON DRINK

2 tablespoons lemon juice
1/16 teaspoon cayenne pepper
1/16 teaspoon ginger (optional)
1 cup water
1/2 teaspoon honey (or other natural sweetener)

Boil 1 cup water. Add all other ingredients and mix together. Drink hot. Makes 1 serving.

ORANGE-BANANA FRAPPE

1 cup orange juice
1 banana
4 dried apricots
1/2 cup plain nonfat or low-fat yogurt

Peel and cut banana into chunks. Quarter dried apricots. Put all ingredients in a blender or food processor and mix until smooth. Makes 2 cups.

PEACH FIZZ

1 cup water
2 tablespoons sugar (or sugar substitute)
6 peppercorns
6 cloves
6 allspice berries
3 cups rip peaches
1 cup seltzer water

Peel and cut peaches into small chunks. In a small saucepan mix water, sugar and spice. Bring to a boil then reduce heat and simmer for 20 minutes. Strain the syrup and cool. Mix with water and serve cool. Makes 4 cups.

PINEAPPLE-GRAPEFRUIT FIZZ

1 16 ounce can pineapple tidbits in natural juice
1 cup grapefruit juice
1/4 teaspoon ground allspice
1/2 cup pineapple juice
1 cup seltzer water

Chop pineapple tidbits in a blender or food processor until fine. Add grapefruit juice, allspice and pineapple juice. Blend until smooth. Mix with seltzer if desired. Serve chilled. Makes 3 cups.

STRAWBERRY SMOOTHIE

2 cups frozen strawberries
1 banana
1/2 cup pineapple or apple juice

Place juice and banana in blender. Blend gradually adding frozen strawberries. Whip until desired consistency. Serve fresh. You can substitute frozen peaches for frozen strawberries. Makes 2 1/2 cups.

SUNFLOWER CAROB MILK

1 cup sunflower seeds
3 cups water
3 tablespoons carob
2 ripe bananas or apples
1-2 tablespoons honey (optional)

Mix sunflower seeds with 1 cup of water. Add carob, fruit and honey. Blend until smooth. Add remaining water. Add additional natural sweetener if desired. Makes 4 cups.

YOGURT FRUIT DRINK

1/2 cup plain nonfat or low-fat yogurt
1/2 cup water
1/2 cup fruit of any kind

Pour yogurt, water and fruit into a blender or food processor. Whip until desired consistency. Serve chilled. Makes 1 cup.

Breads and Muffins

APPLE BRAN MUFFINS

1 cup all-purpose flour (or flour substitute)
1/2 cup whole wheat flour (or flour substitute)
1 cup wheat bran cereal (or bran substitute)
1/4 teaspoon salt (optional)
1 teaspoon ground cinnamon
1/4 teaspoon cloves
1 teaspoon baking soda
1 cup sweet apple, chopped
1 egg
3/4 cup low-fat buttermilk
1 tablespoon molasses
1/4 cup raisins
1/2 cup apple juice

Preheat oven to 350 degrees. In a large bowel mix flour, bran cereal, salt, spices, baking soda and apple. Beat the egg in a small bowl. Add buttermilk, molasses, raisins and apple juice. Mix together the wet ingredients into the dry ingredients. Mix the ingredients until well blended. Pour the batter into greased muffin cups. Bake for 15 to 20 minutes or until the muffins are lightly browned. Makes 16 muffins.

BRAN MUFFINS

1/2 cup whole wheat flour (or flour substitute)
3/4 cup barley flour
1/2 teaspoon baking powder
1 teaspoon baking soda
1/4 teaspoon salt
1/4 cup sugar (or sugar substitute)
1/2 cup wheat bran cereal (or bran substitute)
1/2 cup oat bran cereal
1 cup buttermilk
1 egg
1/4 cup molasses
1/4 cup butter or margarine
1/2 cup raisins

Preheat oven to 400 degrees. Combine whole wheat flour, barley flour, baking powder, baking soda, salt and sugar in a large bowel. In another bowel combine wheat bran, oat bran, buttermilk. Add egg, molasses and butter or margarine to the bran and buttermilk. Mix these ingredients until they are well combined. Add the raisins to this mixture. Then add the flour mixture. Mix the batter until all ingredients are well moistened. Pour the batter into greased muffin cups. Bake for 15 to 20 minutes or until the muffins are lightly browned. Makes 16 muffins

CORN BREAD

1 cup skim milk (or milk substitute)
1 egg
2 tablespoons butter or margarine, melted
1 cup yellow corn meal
1 cup flour (or flour substitute)
1 tablespoon baking powder
1 teaspoon salt (or less if desired)
1-2 tablespoons sugar (or sugar substitute)

Preheat oven to 425 degrees. In a large bowel mix together milk, egg and melted butter or margarine. In another bowel combine corn meal, flour, baking powder and salt. Combine the wet ingredients into the dry ingredients and stir until the ingredients are well combined. Pour the batter into a greased 8 inch square pan. Bake the batter for 30 minutes at 350 degrees or until the top of the bread is slightly browned. Makes 1 loaf.

HEARTH BREAD

4 cups whole wheat flour (or flour substitute)
2 teaspoon baking soda
1 teaspoon baking powder
1 teaspoon salt (optional)
2 tablespoons honey, maple syrup or molasses
1 egg, beaten
1 1/3 cups buttermilk or low fat milk (or milk substitute)

Preheat oven to 375 degrees. Combine flour, baking powder, baking soda and salt in a large bowel. Add natural sweetener, egg and buttermilk. Mix ingredients until a moistened dough is formed. Stir as little as possible. Put the dough in a medium bread pan or shape into a round shape. Bake for 50 to 60 minutes or until bread is slightly browned. Makes 1 loaf.

HEARTH MUFFINS

3 cups whole wheat flour (or flour substitute)
4 teaspoons baking powder
1 teaspoon salt (optional)
1/2 cup brown sugar (or sugar substitute)
2 eggs
1/2 cup oil
1 cup skim milk (or milk substitute)
2 cups berries (fresh or frozen)

Preheat oven to 400 degrees. Mix together flour, baking powder, salt and sugar in a large bowel. Add in fresh or frozen berries. In another bowel mix together eggs, oil and milk. Combine the wet ingredients with the dry ingredients and mix until batter is smooth. Pour batter into greased muffin cups. Bake for 20 to 25 minutes or until muffins are slightly browned. Makes 12 muffins.

HONEY NUT BREAD

1 cup skim milk (or milk substitute)
1 cup honey
1 1/4 cups whole wheat flour (or flour substitute)
1 1/4 cups all purpose flour (or flour substitute)
1 tablespoon baking soda
1/2 teaspoon salt
1/4 cup butter or margarine
2 eggs (or 3 egg whites)
1/2 cup chopped walnuts

Preheat to 350 degrees. In a small saucepan, heat milk and honey over medium heat until mixture is very warm. In a large bowl combine whole wheat flour and all-purpose flour, baking powder and salt. Add liquid mixture and and combine. Add butter and margarine and eggs and continue beating the mixture until it is well blended. Mix in nuts. Pour bread batter into two lightly greased medium sized bread pans. Bake batter for 45 to 60 minutes or until the bread is lightly browned. Makes 2 loafs.

OATBRAN MUFFINS

2 1/2 cups oat bran

1 1/2 teaspoons cinnamon
1 tablespoon baking powder
1 cup nonfat milk
3/4 cup apple juice concentrate
1 medium-sized apple
1/4 cup raisins
2 egg whites
1 teaspoon butter (or butter substitute)

Preheat oven to 350 degrees. Peel, core and grate the apple. Mix oat bran, cinnamon, and baking powder in a large bowl. Pour in milk, apple juice concentrate, apple, raisins, egg whites and butter. Mix until well blended. Place 2 tablespoons of mixture into greased muffin tins. Bake for 20 to 30 minutes or until muffins are lightly browned. Serve hot or cold. Makes 12 servings.

OATMEAL BISCUITS

1 1/2 cup flour (or flour substitute)
1 tablespoon baking powder
1 teaspoon salt (or less if desired)
1/3 cup shortening
1/2 cup uncooked quick rolled oats
2/3 cup skim milk (or milk substitute)

Preheat oven to 450 degrees. In a large bowel mix together flour, baking powder and salt. Cut in the shortening into the mixture until well blended. Mix in the oats. Add the milk and combine mixture until it is well blended. Knead the dough about 10 or 20 times. Roll the dough to about 1/2 inch thickness. Using a 2 inch round cutter cut the biscuits until the dough is used up. Place the dough on an ungreased cookie sheet. Bake for 8 to 10 minutes or until the biscuits are lightly browned. Makes 12 biscuits.

RAISIN BRAN MUFFINS

2 1/4 cup uncooked oat bran cereal
1/4 cup raisins
2 teaspoons baking powder
1/2 teaspoon salt (optional)
3/4 cup skim milk (or milk substitute)
1/3 cup honey

2 eggs
1 tablespoon vegetable oil

Preheat oven to 425 degrees. In a large bowel combine oat bran cereal, raisins, baking powder and salt. In another bowl combine the milk, honey, eggs and vegetable oil. Combine the ingredients until they are well mixed. Add the wet ingredients to the dry ingredients. Pour the batter into lightly greased muffin cups. Bake for 15 to 20 minutes or until muffins are lightly browned. Makes 16 muffins.

Dessert

BANANA MOUSSE

3 medium sized ripe bananas
1/4 cup partly skimmed ricotta cheese
3 tablespoons skim milk
1 pinch ground nutmeg

Peel and place bananas in a heavy plastic bag. Freeze for at least 6 hours. Remove from freezer and cut each into 5 or 6 pieces. Place bananas in a large bowl. Add other ingredients and mix until well blended. Make sure mixture is smooth and creamy. May mix in a blender or food processor. Serve chilled. Makes 3 servings.

CARROT CAKE

1 1/2 cups flour (or flour substitute)
1 1/2 cups finely shredded carrots
3/4 cup honey
1/2 cup raisins
1/2 cup walnuts
1 teasoon baking soda
1/2 cup butter
2 eggs
1 teaspoon cinnamon
1/2 teaspoon salt
1 teaspoon vanilla

Preheat oven to 350 degrees. In a large bowl mix together honey, eggs and butter until smooth. Add flour, baking soda, cinnamon, salt and vanilla. Add carrots, raisins and nuts. Stir mixture until all ingredients are well blended. Pour into medium sized bread pan. Bake for 45 to 60 minutes or until edges of cake are lightly browned. Makes 8 servings.

CHUTNEY

3 medium sized tart green apples
1 medium onion

1/2 cup chopped dried figs
1/4 cup raisins
1 cup cider vinegar
1 6 ounce apple juice concentrate, undiluted
1 teaspoon onion powder
1/2 teaspoon ground mustard
1/2 teaspoon chili powder
1 1/2 teaspoons ground ginger
1/4 teaspoon cayenne pepper
1 tablespoon pickling spices

Peel, core and dice tart green apples. Peel and dice medium onion. Put pickling spices in a tied cheesecloth bag. Combine all ingredients in a large saucepan. Bring to a boil. Reduce heat and simmer slowly uncovered for 2 hours. Cool to room temperature. Remove and discard spice bag. Store covered in the refrigerator. Makes 8 servings.

ENERGY BARS

3 cups granola or rolled oats
1 cup protein powder
1/2 cup coconut
1/2 cup sunflower seeds
1/2 cup butter (or butter substitute)
1 cup peanut butter
1/2 cup honey

Mix dry ingredients in a large bowl. Melt butter in saucepan and mix in honey and peanut butter. Add liquid to dry ingredients. Press in a small pyrex dish, let cool and cut into squares. You can substitute raisins, nuts, dates or other natural ingredients. Makes 12 servings.

FRUIT COCKTAIL

1 cup fresh seedless green grapes
1 cup orange, cut into sections
1 cup pineapple chunks
2 ripe bananas, sliced into small chunks
1 cup pears, sliced into chunks
1/2 cup strawberries, sliced

Use fresh fruit that is in season. Prepare fruit as outlined. Use a minimum of three different kinds of fruit. Use other fresh fruit if desired. Mix all ingredients in a large bowl. Pour into small dishes. Spoon over sauce of fruit. Makes 6 servings.

FRUIT FLAN

1/2 cup apple juice concentrate
1/2 teaspoon cinnamon
3 tablespoons cornstarch
1/4 cup water
2 1/2 cups skim milk
1 egg white
1 teaspoon vanilla
1 teaspoon finely grated lemon rind
1 fresh sliced fruit (optional)

Mix 1/4 cup apple juice concentrate with the cinnamon. Heat under medium heat until cinnamon is dissolved. Set aside. Blend cornstarch with the water until it is dissolved. Mix together apple juice concentrate, milk, egg whites, vanilla and lemon rind into a medium saucepan. Add the cornstarch mixture and cook over medium heat, stirring constantly until thickened. Bring mixture to a rolling boil then reduce heat. coat six sherbet glasses with the apple juice and cinnamon mixture. Put the thickened custard into the coated sherbet glasses and refrigerate for 2 hours. Garnish with fresh fruit slices and serve chilled. Makes 6 servings.

FRUIT PUDDING

12 cups water
1 cup seedless raisins
1 cup apricots
1 cup sugar (or sugar substitute)
2 cups prunes
1 cup dried apples
1 cup cranberries
1/2 cup flour (or flour substitute)

Cut apricots into quarters. Remove stones from prunes. Put all fruit except cranberries into a large bowl with 11 cups water. Cook cranberries separately in 1 cup water. Mash and strain cranberries into other fruit. Boil all fruit under low to medium heat until fruit is soft. Using some of the cooled fruit juice make a thin paste with the flour and pour back into the pot, stirring constantly. On low heat cook the mixture for 45 minutes, stirring constantly so the fruit does not fall to the bottom of the pot. After this time set the pot in the oven at medium heat for 45 minutes. Serve cool or hot. Makes 8 servings.

GINGER BAKED APPLES

4 medium-sized apples
2 tablespoons chopped almonds or walnuts
1 tablespoon currants
3 teaspoons chopped candied ginger
1 1/2 tablespoons lemon juice
2/3 cup maple syrup
1 cup nonfat yogurt
1 teaspoon vanilla extract

Preheat oven to 350 degrees. Add vanilla to nonfat yogurt and set aside. Peel and remove the tops of the apples. Set the apples in a large bowl so that the apples do not touch each other. In a small cavity in each apple add nuts, currants and candied ginger. Mix the lemon juice and maple syrup and pour into the cavities and around the apples. Bake the apples for 30 to 40 minutes or until lightly browned. Remove from the oven and let apples cool. Place each apple in a separate bowl, pour the maple sauce over the apples and top with 2 tablespoons of vanilla yogurt. Makes 4 servings.

GINGER SNAPS

1 cup firmly packed brown sugar
3/4 cup vegetable oil
1/4 cup molasses
1 egg
1 1/2 cups all-purpose flour (or wheat substitute)
1 1/2 cups rice bran
2 teaspoons baking soda
1 teaspoon ground cinnamon
1 teaspoon ground ginger
1/2 teaspoon ground cloves
3 tablespoons sugar (or sugar substitute)

Preheat oven to 375 degrees. Combine brown sugar, oil, molasses and egg in a large mixer bowl. Beat until will mixed. Combine flour, bran, baking soda, cinnamon, ginger and cloves. Add the molasses mixture and mix on low speed for one minute or until thoroughly blended. Form into 1-inch balls. Roll in granulated sugar and place on greased cookies sheet. Bake for 6 to 8 minutes. Makes about 2 dozen cookies.

LEMON MOUSSE

3 tablespoons lemon juice
4 cups nonfat or low-fat yogurt
1/2 teaspoon grated lemon peel
1 tablespoon plain gelatin
3 tablespoons semi-sweet chocolate shavings

Add 3 tablespoons of lemon juice to 4 cups nonfat yogurt. Add sugar and grated lemon peel to lemon yogurt. Dissolve the gelatin in the lemon juice and add to the yogurt mixture. Chill and serve with chocolate shavings. Makes 4 servings

TAPIOCA PUDDING

3 tablespoons quick-cooking tapioca
1/3 cup sugar(or sugar substitute)
2 large egg whites
2 3/4 cups skim milk (or milk substitute)
3/4 teaspoon vanilla extract
1 pinch ground nutmeg
1/4 cup slivered almonds

Lightly beat 2 large egg whites. Mix tapioca, sugar, egg whites and milk and let stand for 5 minutes. Bring mixture to a boil over medium heat, stirring constantly. Remove from heat and stir in vanilla and nutmeg. Cover with plastic wrap and let stand at room temperature for 2o minutes. Stir and pour into individual serving dishes. Garnish with 1 tablespoon of slivered almonds per serving. Serve warm or chilled. Makes 4 servings.

Entrees and Main Dishes

BAKED SALMON

1 fresh salmon
2 large onions
1 cup mayonnaise (or mayonnaise substitute)
1 package onion soup mix

Preheat oven to 350 degrees. Slice onions. In a small bowl mix onions, mayonnaise and soup mix. Spread evenly over salmon. Cover with foil. Bake for 30 minutes or until salmon is cooked. Makes 4 servings.

MEAT LOAF

1 1/2 pounds ground beef (or tofu if desired)
1 crushed clove garlic
1 medium-sized tomato
1/2 cup tomato juice
1 medium-sized onion
1 stalk of celery
1/2 medium-sized green pepper
1 medium-sized carrot
1 egg
1/2 teaspoon salt (optional)
1/2 teaspoon pepper

Preheat oven to 350 degrees. Slice tofu into small bite-sized chunks. Finely chop tomato, onion, celery and green pepper. In a small saucepan mix tomato and juice and garlic. Saute under low-medium heat for 10 minutes. In a large bowl mix vegetables and tomatoes. Add in tofu or ground beef. Mix until well blended. Form mixture into a loaf and place into a medium-sized bread ban. Add salt and pepper. Bake for 50 to 60 minutes. Garnish with chopped parsley. Makes 4 servings.

RATATOUILLE

1 medium-sized eggplant
6 medium-sized zucchini

2 medium-sized green pepper
2 large onions
4 large tomatoes
1 clove minced garlic
1 cup minced parsley
1 teaspoon oregano
1 teaspoon low-sodium soy sauce

Preheat oven to 350 degrees. Peel and cut eggplant in small bite-sized cubes. Slice zucchini, green pepper and onions into small pieces. Cut tomatoes in small chunks. Combine all vegetables into a large bowl. Add spices. Mix until well blended. Place in a medium-sized casserole dish. Bake covered for 1 1/2 hours. During the first hour it may be necessary to baste the dish with some water. Uncover and bake for 1/2 hour. Bake until vegetables are tender. Avoid burning the vegetables. Serve hot or cold. Makes 8 servings.

SPANISH RICE

1 cup onion
1 clove minced garlic
1 cup pepper
1/2 cup carrots
4 cups tomatoes with juice
1 cup brown rice
1 teaspoon soy sauce
1/2 teaspoon salt
1/2 teaspoon pepper

Wash rice and place in a medium pot. Cook for 30 minutes or until rice is flaky and tender. Set aside. Preheat oven to 350 degrees. Chop onion. Slice pepper and finely shred carrots. Saute vegetables for 5 to 10 minutes or until tender. Add spices. Mix rice and vegetables in a baking pan. Bake for 15 minutes. Garnish with parsley and cheese. Serve hot or cold. Makes 4 servings.

STIRFRY

1 pound firm tofu
2 cups broccoli florets
1 cup chopped celery
2 cups chopped bok choy

1/2 cup chopped onion
1 clove minced garlic
1/2 teaspoon garlic powder
1 teaspoon onion powder
1/2 teaspoon salt
1 teaspoon low-sodium soy sauce

Cut tofu into small bite-sized chunks. Mix tofu with garlic powder, onion powder, salt and soy sauce. Cook tofu in a medium saucepan over low heat for 15 minutes. Cook tofu until lightly browned. In another saucepan mix 2 tablespoons olive oil with 2 tablespoons water. Add garlic then onion, celery, bok choy and broccoli. Saute until vegetables are tender yet firm. Combine tofu with vegetables. Stir until well blended. Serve with alone or over rice. As a variation you can use cauliflower, red peppers or other green vegetables of your choice. Makes 4 to 6 servings.

VEGETARIAN CHILI

2 1/2 cups kidney beans
1 cup bulgur wheat
1 cup tomato juice
4 cloves crushed garlic
1 1/2 cups onions
1 cup celery, chopped
1 cup carrots, chopped
1 cup green peppers, chopped
2 cups fresh tomatoes, chopped
1-2 tablespoons lemon juice
1 teaspoon ground cumin
1 teaspoon basil
1-2 teaspoons chili powder (more if desired)
3 tablespoons tomato paste
3 tablespoons dry red wine (optional)
1/2 teaspoon salt (optional)
1/2 teaspoon pepper
3 tablespoons olive oil (for saute)

Put kidney beans in a bowl and add 6 cups water. Soak for 3 to 4 hours. Add 1 teaspoon salt and extra water if necessary and simmer under low-medium heat for 1 hour or until beans are tender. Chop onions, celery, carrots, green peppers and tomatoes. Pour tomato juice in a medium pot. Bring to a boil. Add bulgur. Cover and let stand for at least 1 hour. Saute onions and garlic with olive oil in a large saucepan. Add other vegetables. Continue to saute until vegetables are tender. Add spices. Combine all ingredients in a large bowl. Stir until well blended. Heat over low heat. Serve hot. Garnish with cheese and chopped parsley. Makes 8 servings.

VEGETARIAN CHOW MEIN

4 cups chow mein noodles
2 cups celery, chopped
1/2 head of small cabbage, chopped
1 green pepper, sliced
1 cucumber, sliced
1/2 cup onions, sliced
1 cup bean sprouts
1 cup mushrooms, sliced
1 cup cauliflower, in small florets
1/4 cup water (or juice from mushrooms)
1 tablespoon cornstarch
1 teaspoon low-sodium soy sauce
1 teaspoon salt (optional)
1 teaspoon sugar (or sugar substitute)

Preheat oven to 350 degrees. Chop celery and cabbage. Slice green pepper, cucumber, onion and mushrooms. Saute celery in a small amount of oil or butter for 5 minutes. Add the remaining vegetables and saute until vegetables are tender. Mix cornstarch, soy sauce, sugar and water until well blended. Pour chow mein noodles in medium-sized roaster. Add vegetables. Mix until well blended. Pour sauce over top of noodles and vegetables. Stir in. Bake for 35 minutes or until chow mein is cooked. Serve hot or cold. Serve with rice on the side. Makes 8 servings.

Fish and Poultry

ALMOND CHICKEN

4 chicken breasts, skinned
1 cup almonds, slivers or pieces
1/4 cup vegetable oil
2 cups onions, diced
1/2 cup water chestnuts
1 cup mushrooms, sliced
2 cups broccoli, diced
1/2 cup peas
2 cups celery, diced
1/2 teaspoon pepper
1 cup chicken stock
1 tablespoon cornstarch
1/4 cup water
2 tablespoons soy sauce

Preheat oven to 350 degrees. Bake chicken for 45 to 60 minutes until it is cooked. Remove from oven and let cool Dice chicken into small bite-sized chunks. Set aside. Blanch almonds in boiling water. Remove and set aside. In a large saucepan mix oil, onion, chestnuts, mushrooms, broccoli, peas and celery. Add pepper to taste. Saute over medium heat for 5 minutes until vegetables are tender. Pour in stock. Cover and simmer for another 10 minutes. Add chicken. In a small bowl mix, cornstarch, water and soy sauce. Pour into saucepan and cook another 5 minutes. Sprinkle with almonds. Serve hot. Makes 4 servings.

APRICOT GINGER CHICKEN

3/4 cup dried apricots
2 tablespoons lemon juice
1 clove minced garlic
1/2 teaspoon minced ginger root
1/2 teaspoon cardamom
1/8 teaspoon cayenne pepper
1/2 teaspoon salt (optional)
5 skinned chicken breast halves

Preheat oven to 400 degrees. Place apricots in a small saucepan and add a small amount of water and lemon juice. Bring to boil then reduce and simmer until apricots are tender. Remove from heat. Pour apricots into a blender or food processor. Add garlic, cardamom, cayenne pepper, salt and olive oil. Mix until well blended. In another saucepan lightly brown both sides of chicken breasts. Lay chicken breasts in a pan and broil for 30 minutes. Reduce heat to 350 degrees. Remove pan of chicken and pour apricot-ginger mixture over top of chicken. Bake chicken for another 20 minutes or until chicken is cooked. Occasionally baste chicken with marinade as it cooks. Serve hot. Makes 5 servings.

CAJUN COD

4 5-ounce cod fillets
1 medium-sized onion, chopped
1 medium-sized green pepper
1 cloved garlic, minced
1 teaspoon butter (or butter substitute)
2 medium-sized tomatoes, seeded and chopped
1/2 cup dry red wine
1/4 teaspoon dried thyme
1/2 teaspoon cayenne pepper
2 tablespoons lemon juice

Mix onions, green pepper and garlic in a large saucepan. Saute over low to medium heat until onions are lightly browned. Add tomatoes, wine, thyme, cayenne and lemon juice. Bring to a boil. Add the cod fillets. Cover, reduce heat and simmer for about 10 minutes or until cod fillets are flaky. Makes 4 servings.

CURRIED CHICKEN

1 cup unpeeled chopped apple
1 cup sliced celery
1 cup chopped onion
1 clove minced garlic
1 1/2 cups defatted chicken stock
1 cup sliced mushrooms
2/3 cup nonfat milk powder
1-2 teaspoons curry powder (to taste)
2 tablespoons cornstarch
2 cups diced cooked chicken

1/2 cup fresh or frozen peas

In a large saucepan combine apple, celery, onion and garlic with 1/4 cup chicken stock. Saute over low-medium heat until onions are lightly browned. Add mushrooms and cook for another 5 minutes. Combine remaining chicken stock, milk powder, curry powder and cornstarch in a small bowl. Pour liquid over vegetables and continue to stir until mixture thickens. Add diced chicken and peas. Cook for an additional 10 minutes. Serve hot. Makes 4 servings.

GINGER FISH

1 cup flour (or flour substitute)
1 teaspoon salt (optional)
1/2 teaspoon ground black pepper
4 teaspoons butter (or butter substitute)
4 teaspoons diced ginger or 1 teaspoon ginger powder
6 fresh lemon slices
4 6 ounce fish fillets (cod, halibut, red snapper or other fish)

Preheat oven to broil. Grease medium broiler pan with oil. Combine flour, salt and pepper on a large plate. Wash, clean and prepare fillets. Dip both sides of each fillet in flour. Place on broiler pan. Sprinkle with ginger and cover with lemon slices and butter. Broil for 5 to 15 minutes or until fish is cooked. Makes 4 servings.

HALIBUT WITH TARRAGON

4 4-ounce halibut fillets
1 teaspoon olive oil
1 tablespoon lemon juice
1 teaspoon dried tarragon leaves
1/2 teaspoon ground black pepper
1 tablespoon sesame seeds
1 tablespoon chopped parsley

Preheat oven to broil. In a small bowl mix oil, lemon juice, tarragon and pepper. Place halibut fillets on a baking pan. Pour liquid over fish. Sprinkle sesame seeds over fish. Broil fish for 10 minutes or until fish is flaky. Makes 4 servings.

HOT AND SPICY RED SNAPPER

4 4-ounce red snapper fillets
1 tablespoon cilantro
2 tomatoes, peeled and diced
1 large onion, peeled and chopped
1 small jalapeno pepper, chopped
3 tablespoons capers
3 tablespoons lime juice
2 cloves garlic, minced
1/4 cup water

Combine tomatoes, onion, pepper, capers, lime juice, garlic and water in a medium saucepan. Simmer over low to medium heat for 15 minutes. Put red snapper fillets in saucepan. Simmer for an additional 10 minutes or until fish is flaky. Sprinkle cilantro flakes over top. Makes 4 servings.

LEMON CHICKEN

4 chicken breasts, skinned and boned
4 tablespoons lemon juice
1/2 cup flour (or flour substitute)
1/4 teaspoon fresh ground black pepper
1/4 teaspoon paprika
1 tablespoon grated lemon peel
2 tablespoons brown sugar
1 medium-sized lemon, sliced thin

Place chicken in a small bowl. Pour 4 tablespoons of lemon juice over top. Let marinate for 2 to 4 hours. Preheat oven to 350 degrees. Combine flour, pepper and paprika in a small bowl. Remove chicken breasts from marinade and flip each side in the flour mix. Place chicken on a baking pan. Mix lemon peel and brown sugar. Sprinkle over chicken. Placed sliced lemon peel around chicken breasts. Bake for 35 to 40 minutes or until chicken is cooked through. Makes 4 servings.

Grains and Cereals

APRICOT RICE

2 teaspoons butter (or butter substitute)
1/2 cup diced onion
2 1/2 cups chicken broth
1/4 cup dried apricots
1 teaspoon curry powder
1 cup brown rice
2 tablespoons fresh, chopped parsley

Melt butter in a medium saucepan. Add the onion and saute until soft and lightly browned. Chop dried apricots into small pieces. Add chicken broth, apricots and curry powder. Bring mixture to a boil then remove from heat. Add rice to a medium pot with 2 1/4 cups water. Boil rice for at least 30 minutes or until all water is absorbed and rice is light and fluffy. Add rice to liquid mixture, cover, reduce the heat and simmer for 15 minutes. Stir in chopped parsley and serve hot. Makes 6 servings.

BUTTERMILK PANCAKES

1/2 cup unbleached white flour (or flour substitute)
1/4 cup whole wheat flour (or flour substitute)
1/2 teaspoon baking powder
1/2 teaspoon baking soda
1/2 cup nonfat buttermilk
1 egg white
2 teaspoons olive oil

In a large bowl combine flour, baking soda and baking powder. Lightly beat egg white. Mix in buttermilk, skim milk and oil. Add liquid to flour mixture. Mix lighlty. Avoid overmixing ingredients. Lightly grease hot griddle or skillet with butter or oil. For each pancake spread a large tablespoon of batter on the griddle. When the pancake solidifies and the edges come away from the griddle turn the pancake over. The bottom of the pancake should be golden brown. Cook until both sides are golden brown. Makes 4 servings.

GRANOLA

1 cup vegetable oil
1 1/2 cup honey
5 cups oats
1 cup sliced almonds or walnuts
1 cup sunflower seeds
1 cup coconut
1/2 cup wheat germ
1/2 cup soy flour
1/4 cup bran
1/2 cup powdered milk
1/4 cup sesame seeds

Preheat oven to 250 degrees. Pour honey and oil into a medium saucepan. Warm under medium heat until mixture is thin. Combine dry ingredients in a large bowl. Add liquid mixture to dry mixture. Blend thoroughly. Spread onto 2 cookie sheets. Bake in oven for 45 minutes. Stir granola every 5 minutes. Remove granola after 45 minutes or until lightly browned. Allow to cool. Store in an airtight container. Dried fruits such as raisins, dates, apricots may be added after baking. Makes 16 servings.

IMMUNE SUPPORT BREAKFAST

2 cups rolled grains
1 cup oat bran
1/4 cup dried fruit
1/2 cup raw sunflower seeds
1/2 cup unsalted nuts
1/2 cup lecithin granules
1/2 cup flaxseed
1/2 cup ground milk thistle seeds

Grind nuts, seeds and other ingredients that are too coarse. Mix all ingredients in a large bowl. Before serving soak ingredients for at least 20 minutes with water, milk or milk substitute. To increase protein value add yogurt or tofu to cereal. Makes 8 servings.

MILLET

1 cup dried millet
4 cups water

1/2 teaspoon salt

Put dry millet, water and salt into a crockpot and cover. Set temperature gauge on low and cook overnight for about 8 hours. Serve hot in the morning. Add dates, raisins or other fruits before serving. Makes 4 servings.

MUESLI

1 unpeeled apple
1 banana
2 tablespoons raisins
1/2 cup rolled oats
2 tablespoons wheat germ
1 teaspoon bran
1/2 cup yogurt
1 tablespoon chopped walnuts
4 chopped almonds

Cube unpeeled apple and slice banana into a medium sized bowl. Sprinkle with raisins, oats, wheat germ and bran. Spoon yogurt over top. Sprinkle with chopped nuts and serve. Makes 1 serving.

NUT BREAD

1 3/4 cups all purpose flour (or flour substitute)
1/2 cup granulated sugar (or sugar substitute)
3 teaspoons baking powder
1/2 teaspoon salt
1 cup finely chopped nuts
1 egg
1 1/4 milk (or milk substitute)
1/4 cup vegetable oil

Preheat oven to 350 degrees. Mix flour, sugar, baking powder and salt. Stir in finely chopped nuts. Beat together egg, milk and oil. Add liquid to dry mixture. Beat for about one minute until batter is blended. Grease a medium-sized pan. Pour batter into prepared pan. Bake in the oven for 60 minutes or until nut bread is golden brown. Makes 4 to 6 servings.

OATMEAL PANCAKES

1/4 cup rolled oats
1/4 cup nonfat buttermilk
1/2 teaspoon baking soda
1/4 cup whole wheat flour (or flour substitute)
2 teaspoons apple juice concentrate
1/2 teaspoon vanilla
1 egg white

Chop the rolled oats coarsely in a blender or food processor. Combine rolled oats with buttermilk in a medium boal. Let stand for a few minutes. Add all other ingredients to the mixture and blend until well mixed. Cook on a nonstick griddle or skillet under medium heat. Use 1/4 cup batter for each pancake. Makes 2 servings.

ORIENTAL RICE

2 teaspoons minced ginger
2 cloves crushed garlic
1/2 cup defatted chicken stock
3 tablespoons sodium reduced soy sauce
3 cups mushrooms
2 cups bok choy
1 cup green pepper
1 cup carrots
1 cup water chestnuts (optional)
4 cups cooked brown rice
1 cup green onions
1 1/2 teaspoons toasted sesame seeds

Slice mushrooms, bok choy and water chestnuts. Dice pepper and carrots. Saute ginger and garlic in 1/4 cup chicken stock and soy sauce. Add mushrooms, bok choy, pepper, carrots, water chestnuts and rice. Cook vegetables until tender. Add more chicken stock as needed. Add green onion and sesame seeds. Makes 10 servings.

PASTA PRIMAVERA

3 cups broccoli florets
1/2 pound fresh mushrooms
2 small zucchinis

1 tablespoon olive oil
3 cloves crushed garlic
2 cups tomatoes
8 ounces fettuccine
2 tablespoons grated parmesan cheese
1/2 teaspoon dried black pepper

Sauce:
3/4 cup skim milk (or milk substitute)
3 tablespoons nonfat butter granules
2/3 cup partly skimmed ricotta cheese
1/4 cup grated parmesan cheese
2 tablespoons chopped fresh basil
2 teaspoons dry sherry

Break broccoli florets into bite-sized pieces. Slice mushrooms and zucchini. Stem and cut tomatoes into small pieces. In a large saucepan fitted with a steamer basket lay broccoli, mushrooms and zucchini. Steam for about 3 minutes. Set aside. In a large saucepan heat olive oil over medium-high heat. Add garlic and saute for 1 minute stirring frequently. Add tomatoes and saute for another 2 minutes stirring frequently. Cook until tomatoes are slightly cooked. Set aside. Cook fettuccine according to package directions omitting salt. Drain well. Combine milk, butter granules, ricotta cheese, basil and sherry in a blender or food processor. Pour into a small saucepan and heat over low heat, stirring occasionally until warm. Pour sauce over fettuccine and serve hot. Garnish with grated parmesan cheese and finely ground pepper. Makes 6 servings.

RICE CASSEROLE

8 cups boiling water
1 cup long grain rice
3 tablespoons melted butter (or butter substitute)
2 teaspoons salt
2/3 cup raisins
2 teaspoons sugar (or sugar substitute)

Preheat oven to 325 degrees. Add salt after boiling water. Wash rice well and add to boiling water. When rice is cooked add raisins. Stew lightly and drain excess water. When drained take about 1/3 cup of the boiled rice and spread evenly into a buttered bowl. Sprinkle with about 1/2 teaspoon sugar and 1 tablespoon melted butter. Repeat until all rice is used. Cover and bake in the oven for about 20 mintes. Serve hot. Makes 4 servings.

VEGETARIAN PASTA

2 tablespoons olive oil
6 green onions
1 large onion
4 cloves chopped garlic
1 cup mushrooms
2 celery stalks
2 medium-sized green peppers
1 16 ounce can beans
1 cup water
1/2 cup dry red wine
1/4 cup minced fresh parsley
1 bay leaf
1 tablespoon chopped fresh oregano or 1 teaspoon dried oregano
1 tablespoon chopped fresh basil or 1 teaspoon dried basil
1/2 teaspoon freshly ground black pepper
12 ounces whole wheat pasta (or wheat substitute)
1/4 cup partly skimmed mozzarella cheese

Chop onions, celery and pepper. Slice mushrooms. In a large saucepan heat oil over medium-high heat. Add onions and garlic and saute for 2 to 3 minutes until onions are lightly browned. Add remaining ingredients except pasta and cheese and bring to a boil. Reduce heat and simmer for about 1 hour stirring frequently. Remove bay leaf before serving. Cook pasta according to package directions. Rinse and drain. Serve sauce over hot pasta. Garnish with 1 or 2 tablespoons of shredded cheese per serving. Makes 6 servings.

Salads

BEAN SALAD

1 14 ounce can green beans
1 14 ounce can kidney beans
1 14 ounce can yellow wax beans
1 14 ounce can lima beans
2 medium sweet green pepper
2 medium onions
1/4 cup sugar (or sugar substitute)
1/2 cup vinegar
1/2 cup vegetable oil
1 teaspoon salt (optional)
1/2 teaspoon dry mustard
1/2 teaspoon tarragon
1/2 teaspoon dried basil
2 tablespoons mint parsley

Finely chop onions and green peppers. Drain liquid out of beans. Mix all vegetables together in a large bowl. Combine all sugar, vinegar, oil and seasonings in another bowl. Mix until well blended. Pour dressing over vegetables. Stir until dressing covers all vegetables. Marinate for at least 2 hours. Stir occasionally. Makes 12 servings.

CEASAR SALAD

3 cloves crushed garlic
2 heads romaine lettuce
2 cucumbers (optional)
2 tomatoes (optional)
1 teaspoon salt
1/2 teaspoon dry mustard
1/2 teaspoon ground pepper
1/2 teaspoon worcestershire sauce
1 tablespoon lemon juice
2 tablespoons apple cider vinegar
1/2 cup vegetable oil
1 whole raw egg
2 cups garlic salad croutons

1/2 cup grated parmesan cheese

Rub 1 clove garlic into serving bowl. Tear lettuce by hand into small bite-sized pieces. Slice tomatoes and cucumber. Combine all vegetables in a large bowl. Mix all other seasonings, eggs, oil and 1/4 cup parmesan cheese in a blender or food processor. Mix until well blended. Pour dressing over salad. Mix until all lettuce is covered by dressing. Toss salad and garnish with croutons and remaining parmesan cheese. Serve immediately. Makes 6 servings.

COLE SLAW

1 small green cabbage
1 large carrot
2 cups cauliflower
1/2 cup green pepper
4 radishes
4 scallions
2 teaspoons fresh grated ginger root or 1/2 teaspoon ground ginger
2 crushed garlic cloves
1/3 teaspoon hot red pepper
1/2 cup white wine vinegar
2 tablespoons tamari or sodium reduced soy sauce
2 tablespoons vegetable oil
2 tablespoons sesame seeds or slivered almonds

Shred cabbage and carrots. Cut cauliflower into bite-sized florets. Chop pepper and thinly slice radishes and scallions. Combine all vegetables in a large bowl. Set aside. Combine all seasonings, vinegar and oil in another bowl. Mix until well blended. Pour dressing over vegetables and mix thoroughly. Garnish with sesame seeds or slivered almonds. Makes 8 servings.

GREEK SALAD

1 medium cucumber
1 medium onion
2 medium tomatoes
1 medium green pepper
1/2 cup black olives
1 cup cauliflower
1/2 cup feta cheese
1 cup olive oil

1/2 cup white wine vinegar
1/2 teaspoon dry mustard
1 teaspoon sugar
2 cloves crushed garlic
1 teaspoon salt
1/4 teaspoon pepper

Slice cucumber, onion, tomatoes, pepper, olives and cauliflower into bite-sized chunks. Crumble feta cheese. Combine all vegetables and cheese in a large bowl. In another bowl combine olive oil, vinegar, mustard, sugar, garlic, salt and pepper. Pour sauce over vegetables. Marinate for 1 hour. Makes 4 servings.

MACARONI SALAD

5 cups cold cooked macaroni
2 cups sweet pickles
5 cloves crushed garlic
1 cup onion
1 cup celery
1/2 cup low fat cheddar cheese
1 cup low-calorie mayonnaise (or mayonnaise substitute)

Slice sweet pickles, onion and celery. Combine all ingredients except mayonnaise in a large bowl. Mix until well blended. Add salt and pepper to taste. Makes 6 servings.

ORIENTAL CHICKEN SALAD

4 boned and chicken breast halves
1 carrot
1/4 cup onion
3 cups broccoli
3 tablespoons vegetable oil
3 tablespoons low sodium soy sauce
1 tablespoon dry vermouth
2 teaspoons minced ginger root
1/4 cup chopped walnuts
1/2 pound mushrooms
1 head red-leaf or Boston lettuce

Skin chicken breast halves. Slice carrots and onions. Cut broccoli into bite-sized florets. Slice mushrooms and cut lettuce. In a large pot, combine chicken, carrot and onion. Cover with water and boil until chicken is cooked through. Let cool. Cut chicken into bite-sized pieces and set aside. Steam broccoli florets until tender. Combine vegetable oil, soy sauce and ginger in a medium bowl. Add walnuts, mushroom and chicken. Mix until all ingredients are coated with sauce. Stir in broccoli. Place some lettuce on each salad plate. Top with chicken salad. Makes 4 servings.

POTATO SALAD

6 medium potatoes
2 green onions
1 red or green pepper
4 small radishes
2 stalks celery
1/4 cup finely chopped fresh parsley
1.4 cup calorie-reduced mayonnaise
1/2 cup plain nonfat yogurt
2 tablespoons cider or wine vinegar
1/2 teaspoon salt (optional)
1 teaspoon Dijon mustard
1/2 teaspoon celery seeds
1 tablespoon fresh dill weed or 1 teaspoon dried dill weed
1/4 teaspoon ground pepper

Boil peeled or unpeeled potatoes. Let cool. Dice into small bite-sized cubes. Finely chop onions, pepper, radishes and celery. Combine all vegetables in a large bowl. Combine mayonnaise, yogurt, seasonings and spices in another bowl. Mix until well blended. Pour dressing over vegetables. Mix dressing and vegetables. Toss gently. Garnish with paprika or parsley. Makes 8 servings.

TABOULI

1 cup dry bulgur wheat
1 1/2 cups boiling water
1 1/2 teaspoons salt
1/4 cup fresh lemon or lime juice
1 clove crushed garlic
1/2 cup chopped scallions
2 ripe medium tomatoes
1/4 teaspoon black pepper

1/2 teaspoon dry mint
1/4 cup olive oil
1 cup fresh, chopped parsley

Combine bulgur wheat, water and salt in a pot. Bring to a boil then reduce and simmer for 15 or 20 minutes or until bulgur is cooked. Add lemon juice, garlic, oil and mint. Mix thoroughly. Add scallions, tomatoes and other seasonings. Mix until well blended. Garnish with feta cheese and olives. Makes 6 servings.

TUNA SALAD

3 tablespoons calorie-reduced mayonnaise
1 1/2 tablespoons nonfat yogurt
1 teaspoon curry powder
2-6 ounce cans of water packed tuna
3 tablespoons pears
1/2 head lettuce

Dice pears into small bite-sized pieces. Combine mayonnaise, yogurt and curry powder until well blended. Mix in tuna. Stir in pears. Serve over lettuce. Makes 3 servings.

WALDORF SALAD

3 cups apples, cut into chunks
1 cup pineapple chunks
1/4 cup raisins
1 celery stalk, chopped
1/2 cup green pepper, chopped (optional)
1 cup carrots, thinly sliced (optional)
1/3 cup chopped walnuts
1 cup lowfat yogurt

Cut peeled or unpeeled apples into bite-sized chunks. Cut unsweetened fresh or canned pineapple into chunks. Chop celery and green pepper. Thinly slice carrots. Combine all ingredients in a large bowl except yogurt. Mix until well blended. Add yogurt and combine slowly. Serve alone or over lettuce. Makes 6 servings.

Sauces

BLUE CHEESE DRESSING

1/4 cup crumbled blue cheese
1 teaspoon vinegar
1/4 teaspoon worcestershire sauce
1/2 teaspoon prepared mustard
1/2 teaspoon sugar (or sugar substitute)
2 tablespoons apple or orange juice concentrate
1 cup plain nonfat yogurt

Crumble blue cheese in a small bowl and mash with a fork. Add the remaining ingredients and combine until well blended. Chill for at least one hour until the flavours blend. Serve fresh. Makes 6 servings.

CATSUP

1 cup tomato paste
2 tablespoons lemon juice
1/2 teaspoon dried basil
1 tablespoon water
1 teaspoon onion powder
1/2 teaspoon salt
1/2 teaspoon garlic powder
2-4 teaspoons honey (optional)

Mix all ingredients in a medium pot. Blend until desired consistency. Makes 2 cups of catsup.

CHILI SAUCE

1/2 cup plain lowfat yogurt
2-3 teaspoons chili powder
1 mince, pickled jalapeno pepper
1/4 teaspoon salt
1/4 teaspoon pepper

Combine ingredients in a bowl. Mix until blended. Makes 6 servings.

CREAMY HERB DRESSING

1/2 cup nonfat yogurt
1/2 cup imitation sour cream (or lowfat sour cream)
2 tablespoons minced parsley or cilantro
1/2 teaspoon lemon herb seasoning
1 minced green onion
1/2 teaspoon honey (or sugar substitute)
1/2 teaspoon italian seasoning (optional)

In a large bowl mix together yogurt and sour cream. Mix until well blended. Add spices and mix slowly. Let set for three minutes. Serve hot or cold as desired. Makes 16 servings.

GINGER SAUCE

2 tablespoons fresh minced ginger root
2 cloves crushed garlic
2 scallions
1 hot chili pepper
3 tablespoons sodium reduced soy sauce
3 tablespoons water
2 tablespoons cooking wine
1 tablespoon dark sesame oil
1 tablespoon honey or maple syrup

In a medium bowl combine all ingredients and mix until well blended. Serve fresh. Makes 12 servings.

HONEY MUSTARD DRESSING

2 tablespoons balsamic vinegar
2 tablespoons cider vinegar
1 1/3 tablespoons honey
2 teaspoons Dijon mustard
1/4 teaspoon salt
1/4 teaspoon pepper

In a medium container combine all ingredients and mix until well combined. Serve over fresh spinach for best results. Makes 4 servings.

HORSERADISH SAUCE

1/2 cup plain lowfat yogurt
1 tablespoon Dijon mustard
1-2 tablespoons prepared horseradish
1 tablespoon fresh lemon juice
1/2 teaspoon salt
1/2 teaspoon pepper

Combine all ingredients in a medium bowl and mix until well blended. Serve fresh. Makes 12 servings.

IMITATION SOUR CREAM

2 cups low-fat cottage cheese
1/4 cup nonfat yogurt or nonfat buttermilk
1/2 teaspoon onion powder (optional)
1/2 teaspoon garlic powder (optional)
1/2 teaspoon lemon juice (optional)
1/4 teaspoon fresh or dried chives (optional)

Combine the cottage cheese and yogurt or buttermilk in a medium pot. Add spices if desired. Garnish with chives if desired. Do not mix chives or entire mixture will turn green. Makes 2 1/2 cups.

MARINARA SAUCE

2 tablespoons defatted chicken broth
1 small onion
2 cloves crushed garlic
1 small carrot
3 pounds fresh tomatoes
4 tablespoons fresh basil
2 tablespoons parsley
3 tablespoons tomato paste
2 tablespoons grated parmesan cheese
2 tablespoons italian seasoning

Finely chop onion and carrot. Peel and coarsely chop tomatoes. Finely chop all spices. Heat chicken stock in a large saucepan. Add the onions, garlic, carrot and saute for 5 minutes. Add tomatoes slowly to saucepan. Add the remaining ingredients and simmer under low heat for 1 hour.

Puree in a blender or food processed for a more textured sauce if desired.

OIL AND VINEGAR DRESSING

3 tablespoons olive oil
3 tablespoons cider or wine vinegar
2 tablepoons water
1-2 tablespoons ground mustard
1 tablespoon chopped fresh parsley, basil, oregano, chives or tarragon or 1/2 teaspoon dried spices

In a glass jar combine all ingredients and mix until well blended. Shake to mix ingredients before serving. Makes 6 servings.

ORIENTAL VINAIGRETTE

1 clove garlic
1 cup rice vinegar
1 teaspoon fresh, grated ginger or 1/4 teaspoon ground ginger
1/2 teaspoon low-sodium soy sauce

Crush garlic but do not break apart. Mix all ingredients together and let stand for 1 hour. Strain and serve. Makes 1 cup.

SALSA

2 medium-sized tomatoes
1 small red onion
1-2 jalapeno peppers
1/2 cup coarsely chopped cilantro
1-2 limes
1/2 teaspoon salt
1/2 teaspoon pepper

Peel and dice tomatoes. Finely chop onion. Remove the seeds and mince the jalapeno peppers. Squeeze the juice out of the limes. In a medium bow mix together all ingredients. For hotter salsa leave in the seeds of the jalapeno peppers. For best results serve in one hour. Makes 4 servings.

TAHINI DRESSING

1 cup tahini
1 tablespoon lemon juice
1/2 teaspoon salt
1 1/4 cups water
1/4 teaspoon garlic powder

Pour all ingredients into a medium bowl and blend until desired consistency. Makes 2 cups of dressing

TERIYAKI MARINADE

1/3 cup low-sodium soy sauce
2/3 cup water
2 tablespoons apple juice concentrate
2 cloves crushed garlic
1 1/2 teaspoons grated ginger root or 1/4 teaspoon ground ginger

Combine all ingredients and mix well. Store in a container in the refrigerator. For best results make marinade at 24 hours in advance. Makes 1 cup.

TOFU MAYONNAISE

1/2 pound firm tofu
1/2 teaspoon dry mustard or 1/4 teaspoon prepared mustard
1/8 teaspoon cayenne pepper (optional)
1/2 teaspoon salt
2 tablespoons fresh lemon juice
3 tablespoons corn oil
2 tablespoons water

In a food processor or blender mix tofu, mustard, pepper, salt and lemon juice until well blended. Add oil and water slowly and continue to blend. Scrape the sides of the container and let mayonnaise set for 3 minutes. Use as you would regular mayonnaise. Makes 12 servings.

Soup

BORSCH

1/2 cup onions
1 beet
6 cups water
2 teaspoons salt (optional)
4 potatoes
1 carrot
3 cups fresh or canned tomatoes

Chop onions. Peel and quarter potatoes, dice beet and carrot. Boil all above ingredients until vegetables are cooked. While the above broth is cooking proceed with the next stage of this recipe.

1 cup potato
6 cups cabbage
1/2 cup butter (or butter substitute)
1 green pepper
2 tablespoons dill weed
1 cup modified cream (1/4 cup cream and 3/4 cup skim milk)

Dice potato in 1/2 inch cubes. Chop green pepper and cabbage. Finely chop dill weed. Saute the cabbage in 1/2 cup butter. Remove cooked potatoes from broth. Mash with cream and remaining butter. Set aside. Add uncooked potatoes and green peppers to broth. Boil vigorously for seven minutes. Stir well Sprinkle with dill weed. Keep borsch hot but do not boil because it will curdle. Serve with hot pepper. Makes 6 to 8 servings.

CARROT SOUP

4 medium carrots
1 medium onion
1 cup celery, chopped
2 tablespoons butter (or butter substitute)
1 teaspoon brown sugar
6 cups water
1 teaspoon chicken bullion

1/2 cup sour cream or yogurt
1 teaspoon salt (optional)
1/2 teaspoon white pepper
1 tablespoon chopped mint

Peel and slice carrots. Slice onion and chop celery. Mix vegetables in a large saucepan. Add butter and saute until lightly browned. In a large bowl add water, sugar and chicken broth. Bring to boil, Add vegetables. Cover and simmer to 20 minutes. Remove from stove and let mixture cool. Pour mixture into a blender or food processor and mix until smooth. Return mixture to saucepan. Stir in sour cream or yogurt, salt and pepper. Heat lightly before serving. Garnish with chopped mint. Makes 6 servings.

CAULIFLOWER SOUP

1 medium head cauliflower
2 medium onions
4 stalks celery
3 cups water
2 tablespoons butter (or butter substitute)
3 tablespoons flour (or wheat substitute)
1/2 teaspoon salt
3 cups skim milk (or milk substitute)
2 tablespoons fresh chopped parsley

Wash cauliflower and break into small pieces. Peel and quarter onions. Slice celery stalks. Mix cauliflower, onion and celery in a large bowel. Add water. Simmer for 20 minutes. Remove vegetables from water with slotted spoon. Save water. Put vegetables in a food processor or electric blender. Process until smooth. Blend butter in a large saucepan under medium heat. Stir in flour and seasoning and cook one minute. Blend in milk and reserved water. Cook stirring constantly till mixture thicken and boils. Add pureed vegetables. Mix ingredients and heat mixture. Sprinkle with parsley and serve hot. Makes 6 to 8 servings.

COLD CUCUMBER SOUP

4 medium-sized cucumbers
3 green onions
1/2 cup fresh parsley
2 cloves garlic

3 tablespoons chopped fresh dill or 1 tablespoon dried dill weed
1 quart nonfat buttermilk
1 tablespoon lemon juice
4 to 6 drops hot pepper sauce

Remove the skin and finely grate the cucumbers. Chop the onions, garlic, parsley and dill. Mix all ingredients except lemon juice and hot pepper sauce. Add lemon juice and hot pepper sauce and mix well. Chill the soup for three to four hours. Garnish with sliced cucumbers, parsley or dill and serve chilled. Makes 8 servings.

GAZPACHO SOUP

4 cups tomato juice
2 cups fresh tomatoes, diced
1 small onion
1 cup green pepper, diced
1 cup cucumber, diced
1 clove garlic
1 teaspoon lemon juice
2 tablespoons white vinegar
1 teaspoon tarragon
1 teaspoon basil
1/4 cup fresh parsley
2 tablespoons olive oil
1/2 teaspoon salt
1/2 teaspoon pepper

Dice tomatoes, onion and green pepper into small cubes. Remove skin from cucumber and dice into small cubes. Mix all ingredients in a large bowel. Let chill for at least 2 hours. Serve chilled. Garnish with parsley or paprika. Make 8 servings.

LENTIL SOUP

1 1/3 cups lentils
1/2 cup onions, chopped
1 cup carrots, chopped
2 celery stalks
1 medium-sized green pepper
1 small potato
1 teaspoon tumeric

1 teaspoon chili powder
3/4 teaspoon allspice
1 bay leaf
1/4 cup chopped parsley
4 cups water
1/2 teaspoon salt
1/2 teaspoon black pepper
1/2 cup nonfat yogurt

Rinse off lentils. Cover with water and set aside. Chop onions, dice carrots, celery and green pepper. Mix vegetables in a large saucepan and saute until onions are lightly browned. Pour vegetables into a large pot. Add water, potato, tumeric, chili powder, allspice, bayleaf and parsley. Drain lentils and add to soup. Add salt and pepper. Bring mixture to boil then cover and simmer under low to medium heat for about 1 hour or until lentils are tender. Remove bay leaf. Garnish with 1 tablespoon of yogurt to 1 bowl of soup and serve hot. Makes 8 servings.

MINESTRONE SOUP

1 1/2 cups pea or garbanzo beans
1 cup onions, chopped
4 cloves crushed garlic
1 cup celery, diced
1 cup carrot, diced
1 cup eggplant or zucchini, diced
1 cup green pepper, diced
1 cup fresh tomato, chopped
1/2 cup dry pasta
2 tablespoon salt (optional)
1/4 teaspoon black pepper
1 teaspoon oregano
1/2 cup fresh parsley
1 teaspoon basil
2 cups tomato puree
3 1/2 cups water
3 tablespoons dry red wine (optional)

Simmer peas or garbanzo beans for 2 hours under low heat. Chop onions. Dice celery, carrots, eggplant or zucchini and pepper. Chop fresh tomato. Saute onion and garlic in a large saucepan until lightly browned. Add carrot, celery and eggplant. Add 1 teaspoon salt, oregano, black pepper and basil. Mix well. Cover and cook under medium heat for 5 to 8 minutes. Add green pepper and zucchini if used. Cover and cook an additional 10 minutes. Add water to a large bowl. Pour in vegetable mixture. Add tomato puree, cooked beans and wine. Cover and simmer for 15 minutes. Add tomatoes and remaining salt. Simmer under low heat. Add paste and boil gently until pasta is tender. Garnish with chopped parsley and parmesan cheese and serve hot. Makes 4 to 6 servings.

MISO SOUP

1 large onion
2 medium-sized carrots
2 celery stalks
4 cups cabbage, chopped
5 cups water
4 tablespoons miso (light or dark)
2 teaspoons olive oil
3 thin slices fresh ginger root

Thinly slice onion. Thinly chop celery stalks. Coarsely chop cabbage. In a large saucepan combine vegetables with vegetable oil and ginger root. Saute vegetables under medium heat until lightly browned. Pour vegetables into a large bowl. Add water. Bring mixture to rapid bowl then reduce heat and simmer for 10 minutes. Remove mixture from heat than add miso paste to soup. Stir paste in well. Garnish with chopped parsley or scallions and serve hot. Makes 4 servings.

ONION SOUP

5 cups onions, sliced
3 tablespoons butter (or butter substitute)
4 cups water
1 tablespoon tamari
3 tablespoons dry white wine
1/2 teaspoon dry mustard
1/2 teaspoon salt
2 small cloves of crushed garlic (optional)
1 pinch of thyme
3 pinches white pepper

Thinly slice peeled onions. Mix salt, garlic and butter in saucepan. Add onions and cook until lightly browned under medium heat. Add mustard and thyme. Mix well. Pour onions into a large bowel. Add remaining ingredients. Cook under low to medium heat for at least 30 minutes. Serve soup topped with croutons and grated cheese. Makes 4 to 6 servings.

PEA SOUP

3 cups dry green split peas
6-8 cups water
1 bay leaf
1 tablespoon salt (optional)

Mix above ingredients in a large bowl. Simmer under low heat for 3 to 4 hours in covered pot. Remove bay leaf.

1 cup onion, minced
3 cloves crushed garlic
1 cup celery, minced
1 small potato
2 cups carrots, sliced

Mince onion and celery. Thinly slice potatoes and carrots. Saute vegetables under medium heat with 2 tablespoons oil. Water may be added if necessary. Add vegetables to simmering pea soup.

1/4 cup red wine
1/4 teaspoon dry mustard
1/4 teaspoon thyme
4-6 drops sesame oil (optional)

About 15 minutes before serving add above ingredients to simmering soup mixture. Just before serving add 1/4 cup freshly chopped parsley. Makes 6 servings.

POTATO LEEK SOUP

1/2 cup medium-sized onions
1 clove crushed garlic
4 medium-sized potatoes
2 medium-sized leeks
2 tablespoons butter
5 cups water

1/4 teaspoon pepper
1/2 teaspoon thyme
1 bay leaf
1/2 teaspoon salt
3/4 cup milk (or milk substitute)

Chop onions, peel and dice potatoes and slice leeks. Saute onions, garlic and butter in a large saucepan under medium heat until lightly browned. Pour mixture into a large pot. Add potatoes, leeks and water. Add pepper thyme, bay leaf and salt. Bring mixture to boil then reduce heat, cover and simmer. Simmer mixture until vegetables are cooked. Add milk. Garnish with scallions and serve hot. Makes 6 servings.

TOMATO SOUP

1 1/2 cups onion, minced
3 cloves garlic
1 tablespoon butter
1 tablespoon olive oil
1 teaspoon dill weed
1/8 teaspoon black pepper
6 cups chopped tomatoes plus their juice
1 tablespoon honey
1 tablespoon mayonnaise or sour cream
2 medium fresh tomatoes

Mince onions. Combine onions in a saucepan with garlic, butter and oil. Saute until onions are lightly browned. Pour ingredients in a large bowl. Add dill, pepper, tomatoes and honey. Cover and simmer under low heat for 45 minutes. Five minutes before serving stir in mayonnaise or sour cream. Garnish with parsley and serve hot. Makes 4 servings.

VEGETABLE SOUP

2 cups potatoes, cubed
2 cups carrots, sliced
1 cup celery, chopped
1 medium onion, diced
1 cup canned tomatoes (optional)
6 cups water
1/3 cup brown rice or beans (any kind)
2 tablespoons butter (or butter substitute)

1/2 teaspoon salt
1/2 teaspoon pepper

Peel and cube potatoes. Slice carrots. Chop celery. Dice onions. Mix all vegetables in a large bowl except for rice or beans. Add 6 cups water and boil for 30 minutes. Cook rice or beans separately in 2 cups water. Mix rice or beans with other ingredients. Garnish with parsley and serve hot. Makes 6 servings.

VEGETABLE STEW

2 medium-sized onions, sliced
2 medium-sized potatoes, chopped
3 medium-sized carrots, sliced
2 stalks celery, diced
1 medium-sized eggplant, diced
1 medium-sized zucchini
1 stalk fresh broccoli florets
3 fresh tomatoes, diced
1/2 cup sliced mushrooms
3 tablespoons tomato paste
3 tablespoons molasses
2 tablespoons butter (or butter substitute)
1 teaspoon dill weed
1/2 cup white or red wine (optional)
1/2 teaspoon salt
1/2 teaspoon pepper

Thinly slice onions. Chop potatoes in small cubes. Slice carrots, celery, broccoli and mushrooms. Dice eggplant, zucchini and tomatoes in small chunks. In a large saucepan add butter and saute onion, garlic, potatoes and eggplant. Add salt and pepper to vegetables. Add celery, broccoli and carrots when potatoes are soft. Add wine if desired. Steam all vegetables until tender. Add zucchini, tomato paste, mushrooms, molasses and dill. Cover and simmer under low heat for about 20 minutes. Garnish with fresh parsley and yogurt or sour cream. Makes 6 servings.

Vegetables

ACORN SQUASH

2 acorn squash
2 tablepoons brown sugar
3/4 cup orange juice

Cut squash crosswise, but not through the stem. Clean out squash fiber and seeds and remove. Slice squash into 1/2 inch pieces. Place squash pieces in a large skillet. Combine brown sugar and orange juice and pour over squash. Cover and cook over medium heat for 15 minutes. Turn squash. Raise heat and cook, uncovered for 10 minutes or more until squash is tender and sauce is reduced. Makes 6 servings.

BEETS IN ORANGE SAUCE

2 pounds fresh beets
1 tablespoon sugar (or sugar substitute)
1 tablespoon cornstarch
1/4 teaspoon salt (optional)
2/3 cup fresh orange juice
2 teaspoons orange rind (to taste)
1 teaspoon butter (or butter substitute)

Place beets in a medium pot and cook with water until tender over medium heat. Drain, peel and slice. Finely grate orange rind. In a bowl combine sugar, cornstarch salt, orange juice and orange rind. Cook over medium heat stirring constantly for 5 to 8 minutes or until thickened. Add butter and stir until melted. Pour sauce over warm beets. Garnish with orange sections if desired. Serve hot. Makes 6 servings.

EGGPLANT PARMESAN

1 medium-sized eggplant
10 ounces tofu
1 large egg white
1 cup partly skimmed mozzarella cheese
1 tablespoon all-purpose flour (or flour substitute)

1/3 cup grated parmesan cheese
1/3 cup bread crumbs

1 14 ounce can artichoke hearts
2 8 ounce cans no-salt added tomato sauce
1 6 ounce can no-salt added tomato paste
1 tablespoon olive oil
1/4 teaspoon crushed fennel seeds (optional)
1 tablespoon italian herb dressing
2 cloves minced garlic
1/8 teaspoon freshly ground black pepper
1/8 teaspoon hot pepper sauce

Preheat oven to broil. Peel and slice eggplant in thin pieces. Place eggplant slices on an ungreased baking sheet. Broil each side of eggplant for 3 to 4 minutes or until lightly browned. Be careful not to burn eggplant. Remove from oven and let cool. Reduce heat to 350 degrees. Add tofu and egg white to a blender or food processor. Mix until well blended. Set aside. Shred mozzarella cheese. Set aside. Mix artichoke hearts, tomato sauce, tomato paste, olive oil, fennel seeds, herb seasoning and garlic in a blender or food processor. Mix until well blended. Make sure no lumps remain. Set aside. Layer eggplant slices in a medium-sized nonstick pan. In between layers pour liberal amount of sauce then apply a thin layer of mozzarella cheese and bread crumbs. Top layers off with sauce, cheese and bread crumbs. Break for 45 minutes or until lightly browned. Makes 6 servings.

GARDEN STIRFRY VEGETABLES

2 tablespoons vegetable oil
2 cloves crushed garlic
2 slices fresh ginger root or 1/2 teaspoon ginger powder
1 cup asparagus, sliced
1/2 cup mushrooms, sliced
1/2 cup onion, sliced
1/4 cup chicken broth
1 tablespoon honey
1 tablespoon vinegar
1 tablespoon soy sauce
1 1/2 teaspoons cornstarch

Slice asparagus, mushrooms and onions. Pour vegetable oil into a large saucepan and heat. Add garlic and ginger. Add vegetables. Cook vegetables until tender. In a small bowl mix chicken broth, honey, vinegar, soy sauce amd cornstarch. Mix until well blended. Pour liquid over vegetables. Serve hot. Other vegetables including broccoli, carrots, cauliflower and celery can be substituted if desired. Makes 4 servings.

HONEY-LEMON CARROTS AND APPLES

4 medium carrots
2 medium Golden Delicious apples
2 tablespoons honey
1 tablespoon olive oil
1 teaspoon grated lemon rind
1/4 teaspoon salt (optional)
2 tablespoons water

Peel and slice carrots. Peel, core and cut apples into small cubes. Put carrots, honey, olive oil, lemon peel, salt and water in saucepan. Cover and simmer under medium-low heat for 10 minutes. After 10 minutes add apple slices to carrots and simmer for another 10 minutes or until tender. Serve hot. Makes 4 servings.

MASHED POTATOES

6 medium-sized potatoes
2/3 cup skim milk (or milk substitute)
3 tablespoons butter (or butter substitute)
1/2 teaspoon ground black pepper

Boil peeled or unpeeled potatoes in water until potatoes can be easily pierced with a fork. Remove from heat and let cool. Peel potatoes and slice into chunks. In a small saucepan combine milk and butter. Heat over low heat until butter is dissolved. Remove from heat and pour into pot containing potatoes. Mash potatoes until smooth. Garnish with pepper and serve hot. Makes 6 servings.

ORIENTAL BROCCOLI

1 large head broccoli
1 clove crushed garlic
1/2 cup red pepper, sliced
1 medium-sized onion

3 tablespoons soy sauce or teriyaki sauce
1/4 teaspoon salt
1 teaspoon toasted sesame seeds

Break head of broccoli into small bite-sized florets. Slice pepper and onions. Put broccoli in a medium saucepan. Add small amount of oil or water. Heat broccoli for 5 minutes under medium heat. Add other vegetables and continue to heat. Season with soy sauce, teriyaki sauce and salt. Garnish with lightly toasted sesame seeds. Serve hot. Makes 6 servings.

POTATO SKINS

3 medium-sized potatoes
2 teaspoons nonfat butter granules
1/4 teaspoon garlic powder
1/4 teaspoon ground black pepper

Preheat oven to 450 degrees. Reconstitute butter granules according to package directions. Thinly slice peeled or unpeeled potatoes. Place potato slices on a baking sheet. Dab butter substitute over both sides of potatoes. Sprinkle garlic powder and pepper over top of potatoes. Bake for 15 minutes or until lightly browned. Turn skin over and bake another 5 minutes or until crisp. Serve immediately. Makes 6 servings.

ROASTED GARLIC

4 large heads of garlic
1/4 cup olive oil

Preheat oven to 350 degrees. Peel off loose, papery outer layer of garlic heads. Place upright in a baking dish. Pour olive oil over garlic. Make sure to let oil run between cloves. Bake for 30 to 40 minutes or until garlic is soft. Baste garlic cloves occasionally. Place each head of garlic on a plate. To eat peel off outer coating of garlic clove. Eat with virtually any entree. Makes 4 servings.

SAUTEED CARROTS

4 medium-sized carrots
1 tablespoon fresh lemon juice

2 tablespoons apple juice concentrate
1 teaspoon butter (or butter substitute)
1 teaspoon poppy seeds

Peel and thinly slice carrots. In a nonstick skillet mix carrots, lemon juice and apple juice concentrate. Place over medium heat and saute for about 3 minutes. Stir constantly. Add butter and stir until carrots are tender. Remove from heat. Garnish with poppy seeds and serve hot. Makes 4 servings.

SCALLOPED POTATOES

1 cup onion, chopped
1 1/2 cups defatted chicken stock
1 1/4 cups powdered nonfat milk
2 tablespoons cornstarch
1 tablespoon low-sodium soy sauce
1/2 teaspoon prepared mustard
4 cups potatoes

Preheat oven to 300 degrees. Finely chop onion and finely slice potatoes. Saute onion in 1/4 cup chicken stock over medium heat. Combine all other ingredients except potatoes. Mix well. Place one layer of potatoe in a nonstick baking pan and cover with onions. Then follow with another layer of potatoes. Pour the liquid over the potatoes. There should be just enough liquid to cover all the potatoes. Bake potatoes for 1 hour or until tender. Makes 4 servings.

VEGETARIAN STIRFRY

1 pound firm tofu
1 red or yellow pepper
1 green pepper
1 medium zucchini
1 large carrot
2 stalks celery
2 1/2 tablespoons olive oil
3 scallions
1 tablespoon arrowroot
1 tablespoon soy sauce
3 tablespoons toasted sesame seeds

Slice tofu into small bite-sized pieces. Slice peppers, zucchini, carrots and celery. Slice scallions and lightly toast sesame seeds. Combine tofu and vegetables in a large bowl. Mix olive oil, arrowroot and soy sauce. Pour over vegetables and marinate for 1 hour. Pour into large saucepan and cook under medium heat until vegetables are tender. Add chopped scallions. Garnish with toasted sesame seeds and serve hot. If desired make teriyaki sauce and pour over stirfry. Makes 4 servings.

ZUCCHINI CUTLETS

3 cups zucchini, shredded
1/2 cup onions, sliced
1/2 cup carrots, sliced
1/2 cup green or red pepper, sliced
1 clove crushed garlic
2 cups soda crackers
2 tablespoons flour (or flour substitute)
1 teaspoon baking powder
1/2 teaspoon salt (optional)
1/4 teaspoon pepper (optional)
2 egg whites

Preheat frying pan. Shred zucchini. Slice onions, carrots and pepper. Finely crush soda crackers. Combine all ingredients in a large bowl. Add egg whites as last ingredient. Combine mixture until well blended. Make small patties. Place cutlets onto greased frying pan. Fry both sides of cutlets until lightly browned. Makes 6 servings.

Reading List

Airola, Paavo: How to Get Well, Health Plus Publishers, Phoenix, Arizona, 1974.

Bailey, Covert: Fit or Fat? Houghton Mifflin Company, Boston, Massachusetts, 1984.

Carper, Jean: Foods Your Miracle Medicine, Harper-Collins Publishers, New York, New York, 1993.

Carper, Jean: The Food Pharmacy, Bantam Books, New York, New York, July, 1988.

Diamond, Harvey and Marilyn: Fit For Life, Warner Books, New York, New York, 1985.

Erasmus, Udo: Fats and Oils, Alive Books, Burnaby, B.C., 1980.

Gottschall, Elaine: Food and the Gut Reaction, The Kirkton Press, Kirkton, Ontario, 1986.

Guyton, Arthur C: Textbook of Medical Physiology, W.B. Saunders Company, Philadelphia, Pennsylvania, 1986.

Jensen, Bernard: Foods That Heal, Avery Publishing Group Inc, New York, New York, 1988.

Krause, M V and Mahan, K L: Food, Nutrition and Diet Therapy, 7th edition, W. B. Saunders Company, Philadelphia, Pennsylvania, 1984.

Manahan, William D: Eat For Health: A Do It Yourself Nutrition Guide For Solving Common Medical Problems, H.J. Kramer, Tiburon. California, 1988.

Matsen, Jonn: Eating Alive, Compton Books, North Vancouver, B.C. 1987.

Murray, M T and Pizzorno, J E: Encyclopedia of Natural Medicine, Prima Publishing, Rocklin, California, 1990.

Natow, Annette B. and Heslin, Jo-ann: The Fat Counter, Pocket Books, New York, New York, 1989.

Natow, Annette B. and Heslin, Jo-ann: The Salt Counter, Pocket Books, New York, New York, 1993.

Robbins, John: Diet For A New America, Stillpoint Publishing, New York, New York, 1987.

Ryall, R J: The Digestive System, Penguin Library of Nursing, Churchill Livingstone, London, England, 1977.

Schmid, Ronald: Traditional Foods Are Your Best Medicine, Ocean View Publications, Stanford, Connecticut, 1987.

Index

A

B

C

D

E

F

G

H

I

J

K

L

M

N

O

P

R

S

T

U

V

W

X

Y

Z

Useful Addresses

Association of Naturopathic Physicians of British Columbia
204-2786 West 16th Avenue
Vancouver British Columbia V6K 3C4
(604)-732-7070

or

Canadian Naturopathic Association
P.O. Box 4520 Station C.
Calgary, Alberta T2T 5N3
(403)-244-4487

or

American Association of Naturopathic Physicians
P.O. Box 33046
Portland, Oregon 97233
(503)-255-4863

or

Bastyr College of Natural Health Sciences
144 N.E. 54th St.
Seattle, Washington 98105
(206)-523-9585

Made in the USA
Monee, IL
05 November 2026

67972639R00128